What they are saying about Kids Fi...

"Easy-to-read"

"In *Kids First: Health With No Interference*, [...]
distilled decades of clinical experience into ... easy to-read
book for parents, teachers, health professionals, and all who
share a vision of wellness for generations to come."

—Dr. Christopher Kent
Renowned researcher, lecturer, and representative to the United Nations

"Essential information"

"Easy-to-read book loaded with essential information on how to raise
healthy children. As a parent, the knowledge you have allows you to
make correct health decisions regarding those who depend on you the
most—your children. This book will greatly increase your capacity
to guide your children to a future they so rightly deserve. Help
yourself and your family by reading this book and expanding
your knowledge in the most vital of subjects—your family's health."

—Dr. David Singer
President and CEO of DSE, a Fortune 500 company

"You need this book"

"The world of health care can be a scary place. You need
this book to help you navigate through it successfully and
keep your family healthy without drugs and surgery.
This book reads like Dr. Ogi—warm, friendly and helpful."

—Dr. Tedd Koren
Author of *Childhood Vaccinations: Questions All Parents Should Ask*

"Insightful"

"Every parent has marveled at the miracle of life. Just as a
newborn baby grows perfectly in the womb, as long as there is
no interference from drugs, stress or trauma, the same perfect growth
and development takes place for children after they are born. Dr. Ressel's
insightful and easy-to-read book will give parents the wisdom, knowledge
and confidence they need to raise super healthy drug-free children, naturally,
with no interference! A must-read for every health conscious parent."

—Dr. Eric Plasker
Pediatric Chiropractor, Atlanta, Georgia

KIDS FIRST

HEALTH WITH NO INTERFERENCE

HOW TO RAISE A HEALTHY CHILD OUTSIDE THE MEDICAL MODEL

DR. OGI RESSEL

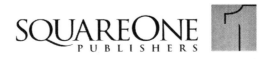

SQUAREONE
PUBLISHERS

Kids First is not intended as medical advice, but as suggested complementary therapeutic regimens, to be considered only if deemed adequate by both patients and their chosen health professional. It is written solely for informationaland educational purposes.

Cover Designer: Jeannie Tudor

Square One Publishers
115 Herricks Road
Garden City Park, NY 11040
(516) 535-2010 • (877) 900-BOOK
www.squareonepublishers.com

ISBN 0-9701110-8-8
978-0-9701110-8-1

Library of Congress Card No. 00-135267
1. Health 2. Medicine 3. Chiropractic 4. Family 5. Childre

Printed in the United States of America

10   9   8   7   6   5   4   3

Contents

To Linda my wife,
best friend, confidant, and soul mate,
who deserves more praise than I have yet realized.

Acknowledgments

My kids—Christie, Adam, and Brandon, who have put up with a part-time father for months, and wondered who that strange man was, babbling incoherently into his computer.

To my wonderful staff who have stood by me and pushed me when I needed pushing.

To all my wonderful patients who have contributed to the book in so many ways.

To all my very important 'lil munchkins for their guidance, love, and inspiration.

To all the Practice Evolution Program doctors who I have taught and who have given me new insight for the new edition of this book.

And lastly, to the College of Chiropractors of Ontario, who have challenged and motivated me and made me realize that the public and the profession would be far better off without their meddling.

And now, on to the good stuff…

My Mission

*To be able to help as many children
in my lifetime as I can . . .
And to be able to train as many doctors
as I can to continue this Mission.*

Introduction

We are in the midst of a revolution in health care. A study, published in the Journal of the American Medical Association, reports that people are seeking health care that is "congruent with their own values, beliefs, and philosophical orientations toward life and health."

The chiropractic profession is at the leading edge in health care reform. As the largest drugless health profession, and the second largest healing art, the chiropractic profession has the vision, commitment, and resources to fill a vital need in society.

In ***Kids - First: Health With No Interference***, Dr. Ogi Ressel has distilled decades of clinical experience into an easy-to-read book for parents, teachers, health professionals, and all who share a vision of wellness for generations to come.

The World Health Organization defines health as "complete physical, mental, and social wellbeing, and not merely the absence of disease or infirmity." This is the goal of the doctor of chiropractic – working to eliminate interference with a person's innate potential for wholeness.

Children are our most precious resource. Regular chiropractic care enables children to experience the joys and challenges of life in harmony with the dynamics of nature. Dr. Ressel has produced this book to empower you with knowledge that will enable your children to enjoy the benefits of a life that expresses their optimum potential for health and happiness.

Victor Hugo wrote, "There is nothing more powerful than an idea whose time has arrived." I must respectfully disagree. More powerful than the idea itself is the individual who has the passion, commitment, and knowledge to make the idea a reality. This book is your guide to making health a reality for generations to come.

-Dr. Christopher Kent

1. Health Care
Not What You Thought?

Before we get into the meat and potatoes of this book, I would like you to do yourself a huge favor. Consider all the preconceived notions that you hold dear about health care: what you or your child may be suffering with; what you may have been told your child has; what you have been told you have; what can possibly be done about these conditions; the role that you may play in your child's recovery; the role that your doctor may play in your child's recovery; the role that a chiropractor may play in your or your child's recovery. Take all of these assumptions, thoughts, and ideas, as well as any other concepts you may have been taught since you were little, place them in a small mental box, and leave them outside. After you have finished this book, you may wish to abandon them forever. If you do, then I have succeeded in my task and you are to be congratulated on having an open mind.

The reason I am asking you to do this is that, in your mind, I would like to create a level playing field. I found that many people I saw in my practice made a number of assumptions about what they have, what they are possibly suffering with and what their children may be suffering with. I find that this type of thinking severely compromised their ability to reason. So…within your mind, I would like to create a proverbial blank sheet of paper, a clean slate devoid of the pitfalls of old ideas, the rubble of old thoughts, the ruins of old assumptions, and on which we can build an amazing structure; a structure that will actually make total sense to you and allow you to take charge of your own health and the health of your children. This is no small undertaking. You would be surprised to learn how difficult it actually is to open your mind to new ideas and new concepts – cerebral constipation comes to mind!

One of the largest quests in the history of the human race has been towards this intangible thing called "Health." One of the biggest obstacles I have found is that most people view health as something they strive for, attain, and once reached, consider it theirs forever.

Most people feel it is then with them for the rest of their lives. Consider the average Earthling getting out of bed first thing in the morning: All toes working, able to stand up – this individual is ready to conquer the world! Right! I hate to burst your bubble here, but *"Health"* is not something you can simply attain, capture and hang on to. It is not a destination. It is a continuous journey. So in the words of Nissan, "Enjoy the ride."

Man has always attempted to achieve good health. Although health has been very elusive, sickness and disease have been very prevalent – and History reveals a number of theories, which have surfaced to explain why people in a society become sick. You will be shocked to learn that this approach to our understanding of sickness is still evolving – with an added twist, however. Yes, money and profit have played a most intriguing part in this evolution.and I just know that you are really shocked to read this.

The first theory, which I call the "Bad Vapor Theory," began in England about a thousand years ago.

BAD VAPORS

Back then it was assumed that people became ill from "bad vapors" which came from swamps and surrounding lands. People believed that these vapors invaded their bodies and were responsible for sickness. In order to regain health, the people of those times felt a need to purge themselves of these bad vapors. I realize this sounds bizarre to us in present day, but don't forget that a thousand years ago this was considered to be the height of science! To stay healthy in those days, people would resort to burning lands and forests, trees and fields to magically rid their environment of these bad vapors. This theory, if you can believe it, has lasted for hundreds of years. Sounds strange, in today's day and age doesn't it?

Wait, this gets better . . .

Although very popular, the vapor theory couldn't really explain illness or produce the expected results. It was eventually abandoned, but not before it was replaced by a more contemporary theory. Perhaps it has a different name, but I am not familiar with it, so let's just call it the "Demon Theory."

DEMON THEORY

People believing in this theory assumed their illness was caused by demon possession. They believed that to be healthy again, one had to rid one's body of demon(s). Again, I know this may sound macabre now, but this theory was highly thought of in scientific circles at the time. It was also during this period that the church was heavily involved in the politics of running most countries.

Therefore, in order to rid people of demons, several "treatments" were employed. The most popular, and probably the one recognized throughout history, consisted of having one's head drilled full of holes to let the demon(s) escape. (I personally have a few relatives that could benefit from this type of care. You most likely do as well....)

As you can imagine, the Demon theory was not very popular as it often lead to all sorts of health complications – most people died following such treatment. Very low on the popularity scale! It was soon discarded with the discovery of blood circulation.

BAD BLOOD THEORY

Medical science soon revealed that people actually had things called veins and arteries running throughout their bodies. These newly discovered vessels carried blood, leading people to quickly replace the Demon theory with the "Bad Blood Theory."

New thinking replaced the Demon theory with the explanation for illness in a society – "bad blood" suddenly became very popular! Therefore, in order for one to become healthy, one needed to get rid of this "bad blood." I'm sure that most of you are familiar with bloodletting: a person's "staff of life" was essentially leaked into a bucket, removed through leaches, etc. Some of you may be horrified to learn that leaches are actually back in vogue whereby in modern day North America, we are actually cultivating leaches for medicinal use. My rationale for writing this is to simply acknowledge that although technology and science may have changed dramatically, the basic thoughts permeating our concept of health are still very Neanderthal. In other words, we have come full circle.

GERM THEORY

I am very happy to report to you that the "Bad Blood Theory" is history. Like the Demon Theory, it too was plagued with public dislike and health complications. You'll be happy to know it was re-placed by a new theory. Scientists of the time, because of the develop-ment of the microscope, discovered new life forms called germs; bacteria, viruses, and so forth. Guess what happened? A new theory was developed. It was called the "Germ Theory" of disease. It was disturbing because it represented new thinking, a new wave in health care. It is still common today, although I am happy to say, it is dying a slow death.

The new "Germ Theory" focused on the fact that now it was known for certain what caused people to become ill – the invisible germ. This thinking was brought about by a number of assumptions, including the belief that germs were foreign to our body and caused illness. So we have been taught that they should be wiped out, killed, and shown no mercy. They should be obliterated in order for humans to survive. Nothing could be further from the truth.

Let's look at the assumptions from which this theory originated.

Your child is suffering from some sort of upper respiratory infection, for example. You find that your child's symptoms may include a raspy voice, coughing, sneezing, and a runny nose, (which may or may not have some greenish tinge in the discharge), slight fever, and a plethora of other symptoms the body may produce. You take your child to the family doctor; he then takes a swab of your child's throat, and 'lo and

behold, finds bacteria in the throat culture. The next step is to announce
to you that your child has "strep" throat. Brilliant! The assumption that
is made, and one that you just bought into, is that your child's health
difficulty has been caused by the bacteria that was in your child's throat.
I love assumptions because they lead to more assumptions and eventually this chain of thought simply falls apart.

Let's take a closer look at this reasoning:

Suppose I took all the patients sitting in our reception area,
or went outside of our Center armed with a Q-tip, and took a throat swab
of innocent pedestrians as they walked by. Then suppose I cultivated that
swab in a petri dish, and twenty-four hours later took another look. What
do you think I would find? You would be shocked to learn that I would
find Pneumococcus, Staphylococcus, Streptococcus, Liberal-coccus,
Republican-coccus and all kinds of other cocci, bacteria and viruses too
numerous to mention. The assumption that is automatically made is that
these bacteria caused your child's health difficulties.

But wait!

If that were the case, then ask yourself this question. Why are all
these people, randomly selected and tested, not sick but my child is? If
Streptococcus was the bacterium responsible for this "strep throat," then it
must follow that anyone having Streptococcus in their mouth and throat would
then develop "strep throat." Right? Wrong! Not everyone does; very few
people actually do. Why is that? What a wonderful question! See, this is an
assumption we have been taught to believe is correct and yet it is absolute
nonsense! Assumptions: they are simply not OK. Let me illustrate further
how demented this thinking can actually become.

Let's assume that you are taking a lovely drive in the country and
on the side of the road you see a dead cat. And let's assume for a moment
that you are totally consumed by curiosity. You pull over to the side of
the road, flip the cat over using a stick, and notice that underneath the cat

there are hundreds and hundreds of maggots crawling in and out. I know this may sound crude to you, but play along with me for a moment.

The normally accepted assumption would be to think, "Aha ... I know what killed the cat! It's the maggots. They're everywhere."

You have just decided that the reason the cat is dead is because maggots somehow infiltrated it, and they caused its demise. That is exactly the assumption that medicine has made with the germ theory. It assumed that just because there are germs found in your child's throat, they *must* be what is causing his/her strep throat, his runny nose or stomach upset, diarrhea, or conditions too numerous to mention that we, as human beings, have fallen prey to. Assumptions – they are not OK!

This type of thinking can be very alarming because it can lead to foolish conclusions. Let me illustrate what I mean. Let's assume for a moment that you are the proud owner of a garbage dump. I know, I know, but stay with me for a moment. And let's assume it is the filthiest dump on the face of the planet. Let me ask you this. What would be the first rodent that would appear in your dump? If your answer is rats, then you are absolutely correct. Now let me ask you another question. What would be the fastest way of getting rid of rats almost instantaneously?

I am not referring to cleaning up the dump, which would be the logical alternative and one that we will cover later, but simply getting rid of the whole population of rats in one fell swoop, overnight. If your answer is rat poison then you are absolutely correct. Rat poison will definitely eliminate the rat population in your dump instantaneously.

How many of you have guessed that I am actually describing the advent of "rat poison" for the elimination of germs? The discovery and use of antibiotics was a truly amazing discovery and very beneficial to mankind. But wait, is it? Let's look at the rat population in your dump for a moment. You had successfully wiped them out overnight and a month later they are back. You then decide that if the rat poison worked the first time then it should again. And it does! The process is repeated month after month and they still are back. You continue to repeat this procedure but eventually, with time, the rats begin to look at the rat poison as "lunch" and it becomes totally ineffective. What I am describing is something that medicine simply trembles at. Antibiotics are becoming ineffective and we are now beginning to create a whole new breed of bacteria named "super bugs." There is little recourse against these "bugs" at the moment. I mentioned earlier that the "Germ theory" of health and disease is slowly beginning to die off. I think it is time for it to die an elegant death. This would be a good thing. In pursuing this "Germ Theory," medicine has adopted an adversarial and combative relationship. The thought has always been "Let's forge ahead and wipe out everything in our way."

Let's think about this for a moment.

How many of you think there are more germs and bacteria on the face of this planet then there are people? If you said "yes," then you are absolutely correct. If we enter into battle on those grounds alone, we will be wiped out in no time. This is why many scientists and researchers are quite concerned that we are creating our very own demise.

I came across a really interesting book recently, entitled *The Coming Plague.* The author suggested that antibiotics have actually advanced the evolution of bacteria by four billion years. How many of you think this is not a good thing? Absolutely! Many patients don't realize that there are a number of bacteria in our own bodies and in our environment that are actually very beneficial and even necessary to our survival. For instance, there are bacteria in your intestines right now that help you digest your food. You can readily see this when you are on antibiotics, for example. When you are on antibiotics, *all* bacteria in your body are killed, even the beneficial ones, and as a result, you tend to get cramps in your stomach, followed by diarrhea, or you are constipated, and your stool color and consistency changes. This occurs because the bacteria that normally help you digest and break down food are killed off as well. Not a good thing!

By the way, for those who need to be on antibiotics for whatever reason, I do recommend you have a natural yogurt or probiotic supplement to replenish the bacteria in your intestinal area. This will aid in your digestion and prevent cramps and diarrhea.

One thing that I would like to add is that most of the time we are able to co-exist with the germs that live inside us in perfect harmony. Pasteur had great difficulties with this type of thinking. He belonged to the outdated model where all germs are "bad" and should be wiped out. (More on this issue in the Chapter on "Dirt".) The prevailing thought of today is that germs suddenly multiply and take over because our body biochemistry has been disturbed and there is increased nutrition available for their growth – and so they multiply.

This thinking fits perfectly with the Chiropractic philosophy of disturbed body function as you'll see shortly.

WELLNESS

This "Germ Theory" is no longer the standard by which everything else is measured. It is now being replaced by a new theory that is beginning to grow at an exceptional rate. It is called … "Wellness." I am sure you have come across this word, but do not necessarily understand what it means. Let me state emphatically that you are not alone. Most people really have no idea what Wellness is all about. Most people's concept of health includes getting up in the morning, looking down at their toes and seeing them wiggling. If they can take a step forward and don't feel bad doing so, then in fact they are healthy – all parts working. They can now forge ahead and conquer the world. That is not health. That is simply survival or existence. It is not Wellness. Wellness means taking responsibility for your health and your destiny. This new movement has spawned a new industry, which includes natural health products, herbs, remedies, spas, fitness centers, etc. All of these methods are presently being used in increasing quantities to capture this elusive thing called health.

There has been a drastic shift, or paradigm, in people's thinking. Not long ago, you entrusted your health to physicians who, you assumed, would do their best to heal you, the patient. This included, in the vast majority of cases, a prescription for medication that would then alleviate your discomfort and/or your symptoms. This school of thought led to the emergence and proliferation of the pharmaceutical industry. The public began to feel, and be taught, that the suppression of symptoms equaled good health. In other words, the public has been taught that when you no longer feel bad, then you must be healthy. Right? Wrong! This is dangerous thinking. It is an attitude that has created the multi-billion dollar pharmaceutical industry.

This present concept of health care rests on the idea of profiting from your illness and your symptoms. It has nothing to do with health care and has everything to do with profit. I realize that some people may be quite disturbed by this line of thinking; however, it is very true. This present concept of health has also generated the idea of arriving at a correct diagnosis for which to prescribe a drug, or a series of drugs to deal with the illness. As a society, we have become obsessed with the idea of treating disease instead of regaining health. We have become a nation on medication – *not* OK!

The pharmaceutical industry has been a leader in defining the role medicine plays in your health. Physicians have been indoctrinated to believe that the more pharmaceutical agents and drugs they use, the healthier the population will become. As a matter of fact, you may be shocked to learn that doctors receive perks and free gifts such as trips, theatre tickets, cruises, dinners, etc., based on the quantity of drugs they prescribe from certain manufacturers. "Better health through better chemistry" has become a motto of Today. Drugs manifesting health—nothing could be further from the truth. This thinking has been supported wholeheartedly by the medical associations of both Canada and the United States to the point where free and clear thinking by certain physicians has been thought of as heresy to the general "party line." (The plight of Dr. Joseph Kropf, and his fight with the Ontario Medical Association is mentioned a little further on in the book).

As Dr. Terry Rondberg, a leader, author, researcher, and friend once said, "as more and more people become aware of the failure of medicine to help them with their health problems, they are turning more and more to herbs and natural remedies to relieve their symptoms and combat their illnesses." In this manner, people are eliminating the dangerous side effects of drugs, but haven't really changed their way of thinking about health. We have been taught since we were children to think of instant health care. This essentially translates into "feeling better." The old "take-a-pill-and-make-it-better" mentality is the biggest health care problem we face in North America."

Many people think that as long as they take some sort of potion or natural remedy that stops their nose running, they are healthy. They believe that if gulping down laxatives keeps them regular, they are improving the condition of their body. The public thinks that since these remedies are "natural," they must be good for them. This is absolutely insane thinking. The basic idea, you see, is still the same. We are searching for a natural *cure* for our symptoms rather than dealing with the fact that they are present in the first place. As a population, we need to stop thinking in terms of treating illness and start thinking in terms of creating *Health* and *Wellness*.

Health (not just the absence of symptoms) is something that we create from the inside of our body. It is not something we can achieve from taking a pill, an herb, or having the latest and newest surgical procedure. If we want to achieve health for ourselves and our children, our goal needs to be: make certain that our bodies are functioning the way they were meant to, normally, with nothing, and I mean absolutely nothing, interfering with that process. That is the key.

Many people don't realize that health is more than just the period between illnesses. It is also not the absence of symptoms. In other words, just because you feel OK, doesn't mean you are healthy. It just means you feel OK and have no symptoms. That's all it means. It does not imply your body is working any better. Health is judged, for example, by how your body is able to adapt to its own internal and external environment. If your body is exposed to some kind of germ or virus, for instance, if it is working normally it should be able to neutralize the affect of that bug, without you even being aware that this is taking place.

This is called health. If your body cannot adapt to such a situation, and handle it on its own, you may begin to get sick. The most amazing thing is that when your body is no longer able to handle a situation, it will actually "talk" to you in a language you can easily understand and listen to; symptoms.

To me, health is like a candle that is lit when you are born and burns brightly throughout life. At the end, it flickers, goes out, ends. However, I have found in my practice that most people do not present with such an idealistic picture. In the vast majority of cases, this is what I would see: The candle is lit brightly at birth, it then has an ear infection, pneumonia, strep throat, tonsillitis, blows out a kidney here, has a heart attack there, liver failure, kidney stones, gall bladder, etc. Often it has to be rekindled and restarted. That's not health. That is merely getting by with as few symptoms and problems as one can possibly avoid.

The medical approach has always been, to prescribe antibiotics, pain remedies and all sorts of drugs to do the job your body was designed to do. People do not realize and understand that those drugs do nothing to help your body regain its ability to perform its functions in the future. In fact, relying on these drugs will actually hinder your body's recovery. (Not to mention all the side effects that are associated with taking them.) There is no pill, potion or lotion on the face of this planet, which can possibly oversee the power of your own body to achieve Health! Most people do not realize that our normal state is to be healthy. Our aim then, as parents, should be to allow our children's bodies to function with absolutely nothing interfering with that process.

And I will cover how to achieve this state in detail.

That's health. It's that simple!

2. Paradigm Shift

How many of you have thought differently about health care recently? I compare this new thinking to a wave; it has been growing in size and momentum and at this point simply cannot be stopped. Let's look at the signs of this new emergence.

Pharmaceutical companies are now placing ads for prescription drugs in general public magazines with the hope that a patient will try to convince his or her doctor to prescribe that particular drug. Even National Geographic has succumbed to this – you'll see many drug ads in your latest monthly edition. The sad part is that many physicians agree to do what the patient asks fearing that if they don't, that particular patient will find another doctor to give them exactly what they want - they will lose a patient and income.

Is this health care or marketing?

Did you know that drug companies are actually rewarding physicians for legal drug trafficking? Many physicians are treated to expensive gifts, trips and Caribbean vacations, for prescribing drugs. In a scathing article which appeared in the New England Journal of Medicine in October, 2004, David Studdert and Michelle Mello revealed that the pharmaceutical industry spends approximately $12 billion annually on gifts and payments to physicians if they meet certain drug quotas.[1] This is especially true in cases of vaccination where the government wants nearly 100 per cent saturation rate. Doctors are often asked to meet certain quotas, and if they do, they are financially rewarded. Is this health care? I don't think so.

On July 10, 2005, I watched the NASCAR races out of Watkins Glen. To my amazement and horror, "Team Tylenol" rolled into the pit. Big Pharma is moving in and replacing Big Tobacco as a sponsor in sports. The object here is to become a household name and synonymous with Health, grandma, and apple pie – an innocuous infiltration of the mind!

---

[1] Studdert David, Mello Michelle, Financial Conflicts of Interest in Physicians' Relationships with the Pharmaceutical Industry – Self-Regulation in the Shadow of Federal Prosecution, New England Jnl Med, Oct 28, 2004. 351.:18 pg., 1891.

Physicians grouping together are another sign. Lessening patient loads, higher overheads, and more insurance and government red tape are turning doctors into administrators fighting for survival in the marketplace.

Wait, there's more . . .

Drug, retail stores, as well as grocery stores are now providing larger areas devoted to vitamin and natural product sales. Market forces are driving pharmaceutical companies toward the manufacture of "natural products." Still others are actually buying up companies that manufacture such products. I am referring to the recent purchase of Quest Vitamins by a large pharmaceutical.

At present, there is a large battle brewing over the increasing use of natural health products. The Canadian government is attempting to regulate the "Natural Health Industry" and make the sale of vitamins, nutraceuticals, and herbal products, etc., a prescription entity. The same thing is happening world-wide: Many are outraged at the European Parliament's March 13th decision to pass the "EU Directive on Dietary Supplements." The directive labels vitamins and natural remedies such as lysine, chromium picolinate and selenium as medical drugs rather than the current classification of "food supplements." In 2005, it will be illegal to sell these supplements over-the-counter in every European Union (EU) country. It will be required that those wanting to use the supplements obtain a prescription from a doctor.

Many believe that the directive has been pushed by the pharmaceutical companies for their own financial benefit rather than the Parliament's claim that it is for the protection of consumers. If consumers can no longer purchase supplements over-the-counter, pharmaceutical companies will eliminate competition.[2] The reason is simple: the pharmaceutical industry has been loosing billions on people who opt to take these products instead of drugs ... And of course, the family doctor has been loosing patients to self-directed health care in the form of natural products that are easily available – and often have better results

---

[2] Health Sciences Institute EU Parliament Classifies Vitamins As Drugs Cosmiverse.com, May 01, 2002.

and no side-effects. From a business perspective this makes absolute sense: eliminate the competition. Get in on the action. Ride the wave. From an ethical perspective – there are obvious difficulties.

If you have noticed the above trends, you are on top of this wave. If you can understand the reason for this shift in thinking, consider yourself ahead of the rest.

DISEASE CARE

There is a strong grassroots movement in Canada and the United States toward a more innate, philosophical, and gentle health care system; a movement that also calls for a non-invasive, and non-pharmaceutical approach. One reasons for this shift is a growing discontent among the public with the delivery of health care in our present system. I use the words "health care" with chagrin; nothing could be further from the truth. Many of you would be surprised that the word *health* does not even appear in many medical dictionaries. Why is that? Because, medicine deals with disease not health. Health is a foreign term. This may sound bizarre to you, but think about it for a moment. If you go to your family doctor and say, "Doctor, I am healthy, what can you do for me?" He/she will look at you like you are an alien, then ask you to leave – not exactly what you had in mind.

You see, Medicine does not deal with Health. It deals with the issue of sickness. There is an incredible difference between those two perspectives. Dr. Patrick Gentempo, a noted lecturer and friend states that "Medicine is actually *sick care* not health care, and when sick care is applied to a society disguised as health care, we end up with a sick society." The medical answer to our health crisis has been to create more specialists, more technology, and more expense. In North America we have the best medical technology on the face of the planet and yet hospitals are always full. The system is failing the health consumer. But (and there is always one of these), the fact that people are sick is actually quite profitable. Are you shocked? Yes, there are huge profits being made from people being sick, and being kept that way.

"You can't solve this problem with the same level of thinking that existed when the problem was created," Gentempo says speaking of our failing and over-burdened health care system.

It is a paradox, yet that is exactly what is happening. It simply does not work. In other words, one cannot do the same old thing in the same old way and expect a different result.

This discontent with our present health care system is causing ordinary people to pose a threat to the authority of the family doctor and the sanctity of the specialist. Enter a patient who is very well educated and asks many questions. Even more threatening is that he/she wants answers to those questions. Most medics are having difficulty providing cogent, logical answers that make sense to people.

MOMS ARE TOPS

You may have not given this much thought, but in North America women, especially moms, make most health care decisions. Think about this for a moment. Mothers tend to make all those trips to the dentist, optometrist and chiropractor more often than dads. When was the last time Dad made a trip to the orthodontist or to the emergency room when one of the kids needed stitches after a nasty cut? Men generally don't even like to take themselves to the doctor. Do you see my point?

I find that women function on a different level than men when it comes to health care. They are very intuitive, well informed and tend to view situations more with their heart, and intuition instead of cold logic. They are not easily fooled and have an innate ability to cut through most bologna and get at the truth. Women pose the greatest threat to the family physician, because they want straight answers in terms of health care for themselves and their families. Can you think of circumstances or decisions in your own life or family where this is true? If so, then you know exactly what I am referring to.

To illustrate the momentum and scope of this shift, allow me to provide you with some amazing statistics. In a study[3] performed by Harvard Medical School, it was determined that in 1991 there were approximately 328 million office visits made in the U.S. to physicians, hospitals, radiologists, gynecologists, and the whole medical machine.

---

[3] Eisenberg, D., et al., "Unconventional medicine in the United States; prevalence, costs, and patterns of use." *New England Journal of Medicine*, Jan. 28, 1993; 328(4) 246-52.

In that same year, there were approximately 425 million office visits made to chiropractors and naturopathic doctors. How is that for a trend?

That same study was repeated in 1997 and revealed that office visits to physicians, etc., had risen to 358 million while office visits to chiropractors and naturopathic doctors was close to 800 million … and the trend is growing. I always smirk to myself when I hear of a new agency formed for the study and development of "Alternative Medicine." Medicine has for years regarded with disdain any profession that was not part of "them." It is interesting to note that the tables have turned: Medicine can now be regarded as "alternative" based on the sheer numbers of people seeking help from doctors like myself.

For those who still feel that my doubt of the medical profession posing as health care is far fetched, the following may be of considerable interest.

MEDICAL ERRORS

Did you know that you stand a seven-times greater chance of dying from walking into your doctor's office than you do from sitting behind the wheel of your automobile? According to the International Chiropractic Pediatric Association, it is estimated that in 1994, approximately 2,216,000 patients who were hospitalized in the United States had serious adverse drug reactions. "Serious adverse drug reactions" are defined as those resulting in death, causing permanently disability, or requiring hospitalization.

Of that number, 106,000 had fatal adverse drug reactions. That places fatal drug reactions between the third and sixth leading causes of death. I excluded errors in drug administration, noncompliance, overdose, drug abuse, therapeutic failures, and non-fatal adverse drug reactions. The incidence of serious and fatal adverse drug reactions in U.S. hospitals was found to be extremely high! Even when the cause is known to be a drug, it is rarely recorded on the death certificate. For example, a stomach hemorrhage might be listed on the death certificate as the cause of death, without mention of the drug that actually caused it. Nice touch!

Therapeutic drug use (not illicit drug use) each year, kills as many as 198,815 people, puts 8.8 million people in hospitals, accounts for 28 percent of all hospital admissions, and costs as much as $182 *billion* dollars.[4]

A scathing article appeared in the December 9, 2002 issue of the Washington Post, and compared the mismanagement and melt-down of Enron, to the Medical profession's inability in reducing the rate of medical errors in hospitals.[5] These errors, according to an Institute of Medicine study three years ago, kill between 44,000 and 98,000 patients annually while injuring perhaps one million more.

The article then goes on to state that reforms are "scandalously slow" and that asking the medical profession to regulate themselves has been ineffective. The article states that the sources of errors are various including, mixing up patients' X-rays, or looking at them upside-down; as a result, they operate on the wrong patient or the wrong body part. Additionally, cleanliness was an issue as doctors and health workers fail to follow basic hygiene procedures such as washing hands or changing gloves, therefore causing infections that account for thousands of deaths a year. The article also stated, "So long as patients have no way of finding out which hospitals are unreliable, bad hospitals will face minimal incentives to invest in the solutions that could drive error rates down. State or federal regulators should require the reporting of errors and should make some of this information public. Otherwise thousands will continue to die needlessly and with no one held to account."

The Lancet, a prestigious scientific journal, reported that medication-error deaths are rising and that one out of every 131 outpatient deaths is caused by medication error.[6] The journal goes on to state that, "patients must understand [the chance of medica errors], and be warned about the potential dangers of prescription drugs."

On the other hand, medical malpractice is the third leading cause of preventable death in the United States. Malpractice is responsible for the deaths of 80,000 people annually – one every seven minutes. This does not include iatrogenic injury – caused by doctors.[7] Every year, close to 180,000 people die, partly as a result of iatrogenic injury.[7] This is the equivalent of three jumbo jet crashes every two days. Twenty percent of

---

[4] American Medical News, Jan. 15, 1996, p. 11.

[5] Washington Post, December 9, 2002.

[6] Phillips, D. P., Christenfeld, N., Glynn, L.M., "Increases in U.S. medication-error deaths between 1983 and 1993" [letter], *Lancet*, 1998, 351 (9103): 643.

all patients admitted to a university hospital suffered iatrogenic injury. Thirty percent of those admitted to a teaching hospital suffered an iatrogenic event, twenty-five percent of which were serious or life threatening. Sixty-four percent of cardiac arrests at a teaching hospital were preventable. Most were caused by errors in the use of medications.

Health care personnel identified 480 patients out of 1,047 studied who experienced adverse events. Of these, 185 resulted in serious complications ranging from temporary disability to death. Forty-five percent of patients suffered inappropriate care resulting in complications or medical injury caused by a hospital staff member. At least 17.7 percent had one serious adverse event, while 37.8 percent of adverse events were caused by an individual. The number of patients who experienced serious events that led to longer hospital stays and increased costs to patients was 17.7 percent. The likelihood of experiencing an adverse event increased about six percent for each day of a hospital stay.

Drug errors not only increase costs but also significantly prolong hospital stays and increase the risk of death almost two-fold. Preventable drug-related morbidity and mortality was estimated to cost $76.6 billion in the ambulatory setting in the United States.[8] The largest component of this total cost was associated with drug-related hospitalizations. The estimated cost ranged from a conservative figure of $30.1 to $136.8 billion in a worst-case scenario.

It is estimated that the annual additional costs associated with preventable [adverse drug events] were $2.8 million and that the costs associated with all [adverse drug events] were $5.6 million.[9]

Several easily identifiable factors are associated with a large proportion of medical prescribing errors. Factors commonly associated with errors in prescribing medications were:

a. Inadequate knowledge or use of knowledge regarding
    drug therapy.

---

[7] Leape, L.L., *Error in Medicine*, Journal American Medical Association, 1994, 272(23): 851-7.
[8] Johnson, J.A., Bootman, J.L., *Drug-related morbidity and mortality. A cost-of-illness model.* Arch Intern Med., 1995; 155(18):1949-56.
[9] Bates, D. W., Spell, N., Cullen, D. J., Burdick, E., Laird, N., Petersen, L. A., Small, S. D., Sweitzer, B. J., Leape, L. L., *The Costs of Adverse Drug Events in Hospitalizations.*, Adverse Drug Events Prevention Study Group, JAMA, 1997; 277(4):307-11.

b. Presence of important patient factors related to drug therapy such as age impaired renal function and drug allergy.
c. The need for calculation of drug doses.
d. Specialized dosage formulation characteristics and medication prescribing nomenclature.

Adverse drug events in hospitalized patients are "countable, dangerous and evaluable events, not just a collection of unhappy accidents that strike, like cosmic rays, in ways that we cannot predict or understand. In an era of constrained resources, it is vital to remember that [drug errors] in hospitals are common, costly and preventable in many cases."[10]

Did you know that a whooping one out of every 17 times a medication is ordered to be given to a hospitalized child, the child receives the wrong drug or dose according to a new study in Journal of the American Medical Association? Potentially harmful medication errors occur 3 times more often among hospitalized children than adults. In a six-week study at Children's Hospital Boston and Massachusetts General Hospital for Children, researchers found 616 medication errors out of 10,778 orders written – an error rate of 5.7 percent. The overall error rate was similar to those found in previous studies of adult hospitals, but the number of potentially harmful errors is 3 times greater among children. The rate of potential adverse drug events was significantly higher in neonates in the neo-natal intensive care unit. "Medication errors are common in pediatric settings, and further efforts are needed to reduce them," concluded the study's authors.[11]

Just in case you doubt me in any way, another report (*Kids in ER face 1 in 10 chance of medical error*) published in the journal *Pediatrics* has revealed that one in every 10 children treated in the emergency room may be the victim of a medical error. The study showed that 10 percent of children going to the ER either get the wrong dose of medicine or are given drugs at an incorrect frequency. Dr. Eran Kozer of

---

[10] Johnson, J., et. al., "Drug related morbidity and mortality , a cost-of-illness model." *Arch Intern Med*, 1995; 155(18): 1949-56.
[11] Kaushal Rainu et al: "Medical Errors and Adverse Drug Events in Pediatric Inpatients," *JAMA*, Apr 2001: 285: 2114-2140.

the Hospital for Sick Children in Toronto and colleagues, reviewed the medical records of 1,532 children treated in the emergency room of a pediatric hospital, and evaluated each one separately to determine whether a medication error had occurred. Children seen between 4:00 and 8:00 a.m., children with severe disease, and those treated on weekends were 1.5–2.5 times more likely to experience a medication prescribing error. Errors were also more likely when a trainee doctor had ordered the medication. The researchers concluded: "Medication errors are a common cause of iatrogenic morbidity and mortality." In other words, people often die because doctors give them the wrong drugs, and children are often the victim of these errors."[12]

And just when you though it was safe to go into the water.....

More than one out of every five people taking part in a health care quality survey said that they or a family member experienced a mistake in a doctor's office or hospital or were given the wrong medication or dose. About half (51 percent) of those who experienced an error reported it as serious. The survey was conducted by Commonwealth Fund.

Speaking at the American Academy of Orthopaedic Surgeons' (AAOS) Orthopaedics Update 2002 web conference, James H. Herndon, M.D., AAOS first vice president and professor of orthopaedic surgery at Harvard Medical School and chairman, department of orthopaedic surgery at Massachusetts General, and Brigham Women's Hospital in Boston, stated: "As the analysis from the Commonwealth Survey says, the American health care system is unparalleled in technological sophistication and medical advancements, yet we fall far short of the ideal when it comes to the safety and efficacy of our health care services."

Falling "short of the ideal" may be a considerable understatement.

The Institute of Medicine's (IOM) widely circulated 1999 report "To Err is Human," estimates that these medical errors cost the United States approximately $29 billion each year.[13]

---

[12] Kozer, Eran; "Variables Associated With Medication Errors in Pediatric Emergency Medicine," *Journal of Pediatrics*, Vol 110, No 4, Oct. 4, 2002, pp 737-742.

[13] "Patient safety – doctors and patients together can prevent medical errors" American Academy of Orthopaedic Surgeons, October 17, 2002.

As I mentioned earlier, prescription drug adverse reactions are a leading cause of death in North America. Every year, approximately 200,000 people die from prescription drug reactions; this from properly prescribed medication, at the proper dosage, to the right patient, for the right condition, and at the right time. Another 80,000 people die from medical malpractice (and although approximately three million people per year are affected, only a fraction goes ahead in launching a formal legal proceeding). In comparison, only a "mere" 41,000 people per year die in auto accidents.[14] Let me ask you this: what is wrong with our focus on the supposed "drug war" we teach our children about, when over 200,000 people die each year from legally prescribed drugs and only 20,000 people die from illegal drug use? What I find amazing is that people still find this difficult to believe. I think this must have something to do with intellectual constipation! The sale of pharmaceuticals is a multibillion-dollar industry in North America. Most people wonder what the Federal Drug Administration is doing – probably approving another drug – and how many more people will die from this one? You don't believe me? Please read on.

In 1992, the U.S. Food and Drug Administration began receiving much of its income from the companies it's supposed to regulate: the drug manufacturers. At the time – and ever since – critics said the plan, called the Prescription Drug User Fee Act (PDUFA), is like asking the wolf to guard the sheep. When their salaries come from the drug makers, there can be little assurance that FDA officials will put public safety first.

Time has proven the critics right. A new government report shows that since the PDUFA was implemented, an increased number of newly approved drugs have been found to be unsafe and have been withdrawn. (Celebrex, Vioxx, etc.) And while I'm speaking of Vioxx, a May 28, 2005, article in the Toronto Star reported that the risk of heart attacks was 400 percent greater in patients who consumed Vioxx. A subsequent article in December, 2005, in that same paper, stated that to deal with the rising onslaught of civil lawsuits over the side effects of Vioxx, will take roughly just over 3,000 years.[15]

This isn't the first time that flaws in the FDA policy have been

---

[14] www.drugawareness.org
[15] Toronto Star, Arthritis Drug May Lead to Heart risks, Study Says. May 28, 2005.

exposed. In 1998, the health consumer advocacy group, Public Citizen, conducted a survey of the physicians who review new drug applications – the people who are supposed to be the final judges as to whether a drug is approved or not. It found that, in the previous three years, the reviewing physicians had opposed the approval of 27 drugs – yet all got the go-ahead from the FDA! The report documented how physicians were precluded from presenting data adverse to the drugs they were reviewing at FDA Advisory Committee meetings.

The General Accounting Office's (GAO) conclusions confirm the major public health consequences of PDUFA, which introduced private money, and therefore influence, into the drug approval process, creating a massive conflict of interest. One result of PDUFA has been the diversion of agency funds to the review process from other areas, including post-marketing safety surveillance.

FDA approvals of unsafe drugs have led to unnecessary patient deaths and illnesses, as well as poor morale among drug reviewers (the GAO report also documents that staff turnover is higher among FDA scientists than among scientists in other government agencies).

"Congress should immediately conduct meaningful oversight hearings on each of the drugs that has been withdrawn for safety reasons," argued Peter Lurie, deputy director of Public Citizen's Health Research Group. "Drug makers have benefited from PDUFA, making millions in profits off drugs that should never have been brought to the market. Congress must adequately fund the FDA's drug approval activities and remove private influence from the equation."[16]
This from Washington.....

"FDA official: Safety system broken down: – Washington/ June 09, 2005 7:11:28 PM EST.[17]

"A top U.S. Food and Drug Administration official says much still remains to be done by the government to uncover the dangers in drugs already on the market. The warning was issued to a medical advisory board in Washington by Dr. Janet Woodcock, FDA's deputy commissioner of operations, the New York Times reported Thursday."

---

[16] GAO Report Backs Link Between Drug User Fees and Higher Rate of Drug Withdrawals, Public Citizen, Sept. 25, 2002.
[17] Safety system broken down:- Washington/June 09, 2005 7:11:28 PM IST AP Newswire

Woodcock, who has been asked to suggest safety improvements because of recent well-publicized drug industry troubles, said the government's safety system needs to be fixed, the report said. The keystone of the current system is the prescriber and that person is the one who decides if the benefits of a drug outweigh the risks for that patient, Woodcock said. This system has obviously broken down to some extent, as far as the fully informed provider and the fully informed patient. She also said physician and hospital errors are major contributors to the current problem.

You thought I was making all this up, perhaps?

Try this. "The Lancet Editorial accuses FDA of corruption: The Lancet has printed a strongly worded editorial accusing the U.S. Food and Drug Administration of being a "servant" of the pharmaceutical industry. The article, "Lotronex and the FDA: A Fatal erosion of integrity," by Richard Horton, focuses on the FDA's February, 2000, licensure of GlaxoSmithKline's drug for irritable bowel syndrome. Lotronex was withdrawn voluntarily by GlaxoSmithKline in November, 2000, after it was associated with five deaths and dozens of hospitalizations (several requiring surgery). According to Horton, the drug company "bought" approval by funneling millions of dollars into FDA research. Horton also claims that the FDA refused to hear presentations from scientists who questioned the drug's safety, and did not pull the drug's license when it first became clear that he medication was deadly. "The FDA is not only compromised because it receives so much funding from pharmaceutical industry, but because it comes under incredible Congressional pressure to be favorable to pharmaceutical industry," wrote Horton. "That has led to deaths."[18]

There are many outspoken leaders who question our wisdom and our national urge to view medicine as health care. One of the most prestigious is Mr. Jon Rappoport, an investigative journalist, who was nominated for the Pulitzer Prize by *Los Angeles Weekly*. Mr. Rappoport has also authored books on AIDS, the CIA, etc. He has

---

[18] Horton Richard, "Lotronex and the FDA: A Fatal erosion of integrity," Lancet, May 19, 2001; 357:1544-1545.

made guest appearances on *Night Line, Hard Copy* and other radio and television programs.

Mr. Rappoport writes, "The medical Cartel is not medical at all. It is concerned with controlling populations. 99.99 percent of the people who work in any capacity for this Cartel do not have the faintest idea about this, they are sincere and sometimes helpful and are always indoctrinated beyond their own rationality." He further states that, "in a very real sense the world is being invented. I have spent the last 20 years uncovering it, who's inventing it, how they are doing it, for what reasons, and what we can do about it." We have been indoctrinated that this is our reality when in fact this image of health, as we know it, has been carefully contrived for the sake of profit. So you see, medicine has been sold to the public as health care for decades. At long last, the amour of this Cartel is beginning to crack and medicine, as an organization, must finally stand up, face the public and account for its inadequacies."

If you are still not convinced, reports in newspapers and TV broadcasts very often exaggerate the benefits of new medicines and drugs and ignore the risks or fail to disclose their costs.[19] The Harvard medical study published in the New England Journal of Medicine also examined potential conflicts of interest. It found that most researchers had financial ties to drug companies and only thirty percent would disclose those ties. This study focused on 207 news reports done on new drugs released. Forty percent did not offer any analysis of the drugs benefits, leaving the public totally unaware of how to judge the value of a drug. The study also found that benefits are grossly exaggerated. As an illustration, the study reported on a new 1996 drug for osteoporosis, which was said to reduce hip fractures by fifty percent. However, that figure was found to be grossly exaggerated, in that only two percent of untreated osteoporosis sufferers would sustain a hip fracture. So the new drug would reduce hip fractures from two to one percent in that population only. This study also found that most reports failed to discuss the potential harm of the medication as well as the cost effectiveness of the drug.

This from the July 11, 2005 issue of *USA Today*: "Blindness Warning Added to Viagra." The article explained that blindness can be a

---

[19] Moynihan, Ray et al; Coverage by the News Media of the benefits and risks of medications, *New Enl Journal of Medicine*, June 1, 2000. No 22, Vol; 342:1645-1650

side-effect of Viagra, Cialis and Levitra – the manufacturer quickly pointed out that these effects are rare.[20]

I feel better already – those who lost their vision may not!

And here is the final word on medical studies: A brand new study found that what you were once told was good for you, has turned out to be not so good – there is a surprise! Dr. John Ioannidis reviewed major medical research studies done between 1990 and 2003 and found that the purported results don't hold water in 32 percent of cases. His finding were published in the Journal of the American Medical Association. The sad reality is that millions of patients were affected. And how many of those are on the medical error stats.[21]

These are some of the reasons why people are turning away from traditional medical care and flooding the offices of chiropractors, naturopaths, homeopaths, and other so called "alternative" practitioners. I would also like to point out that I do not consider chiropractic as "alternative." I feel that it stands on its own as a separate healing profession based on a different set of values and principles. In that, and its tremendous success, it has no equal!

The public is beginning to realize more and more that the practice of medicine is essentially "crisis control" and is based on symptom attenuation, changing body chemistry, and fear. It is not health care.

You may be shocked reading this but hang in there for a bit ... I'll give you more food for thought!

The late Dr. Robert Mendelsohn, M.D., a famed and self-proclaimed "medical heretic," put this into an interesting context.[22] "In 1976, physicians in Bogota, Columbia, went on a 52 day strike. The National Catholic Reporter described a string of unusual "side-effects" from the strike. The death rate went down 35 percent." A spokesman for the National Morticians Association said, "It might be coincidence but it is fact." In Los Angeles, the death rate dropped 18 percent when doctors went on strike to protest soaring malpractice premiums. When the strike ended, the death rate once again rose to pre-strike levels.

---

[21] "A Final Word on Medical Studies" Toronto Star, Wednesday, July 13, 2005, pg A16
[22] Mendelsohn, R., *The Medical Heretic,* Chicago Contemporary Books, 1979, 114.

The most striking evidence was seen in Israel though. Doctors reduced their daily patient contact from 65,000 to 7,000 for one month. According to the Jerusalem Burial Society, the Israeli death rate dropped 50 percent during that month."

As if to reinforce the point, an on-going strike by medical doctors in Israel had put a severe economic strain on the funeral business in that country. The dramatic decline in the death rate prompted the burial association to ask the government to approve an increase in doctors' pay.

According to the newspaper, *The Jerusalem Sun*, strike action by doctors in Israel seemed to be good for their patients' health. A survey of burial societies revealed that death rates dropped considerably in most of the country since physicians in public hospitals implemented a program of sanctions lasting three months.[23] Meir Adler, manager of the Shaingar Funeral Parlour, which buries most of the residents of Jerusalem, declared with much more certainty, "There definitely is a connection between the doctors' sanctions and fewer deaths. We saw the same thing in 1983." (when the Israel Medical Association applied sanctions for four and one half months).

Those of you who believe that medicine represents health care may feel quite shocked by this time – I totally understand.

But, let's go on.

A recent study by Dr. Bruce H. Pomeranz, the principal investigator and professor at the University of Toronto, Canada, shed light on this phenomenon. Dr. Pomeranz estimated that adverse reactions to prescription and over-the-counter medications kill more than 100,000 Americans and seriously injure an additional 2.1 million people every year – I feel that he had just scratched the surface of the problem. Such reactions, which do not include prescribing errors or drug abuse, rank as a leading cause of death.[24] Dr. Mendelsohn felt that what is really in true health care is a perpetual doctors' strike. "If doctors reduced their involvement with people by 90 percent, and attended only emergencies, there's no doubt in my mind that we'd be better off."

---

[23] Doctors Strike in Israel: http://www.bmj.conVcgi/content/full/320/7249/1561 British Medical Journal, June 10, 2000.

[24] Journal of the American Medical Association, April 15, 1998.

You may not have considered this, but at best, there are only five viable options available to most physicians when faced with a patient who has a health problem:

    a. Wait for it to "go away" on its own or "live with it." I am sure many of you have heard those words.

    b. Prescribe drugs in the hope that this will somehow minimize the symptoms.

    c. Refer the patient for surgery to remove the malfunctioning or diseased organ or ... other radical procedure.

    d. Physiotherapy.

    e. Experimental options; there are many of these and are the most frightening on this list.

Beyond that, there are really no other options left. I am sure that many of you have heard from your own family or friends about situations where an individual has returned from seeing the family doctor with a statement that "We can't help you and you will have to learn to live with it." I find nothing more degrading and invalidating to a Human Being than those words. I find the attitude insulting and arrogant. Just because medicine cannot help this particular patient, does not mean that another health care professional will have the same finding. As a matter of fact, the public is beginning to discover that this is exactly what has been happening. The patient of today is no longer satisfied with this approach to health. Gone are the days when a patient is appeased with hearing from their doctor "I am your doctor, I know what is best for you, trust me."

The medical associations in Canada and the United States have responded to this shift of thinking in a very predictable manner. The CMA and the AMA policy seem to be very clear, "let's wipe out our opposition." This is particularly true of the chiropractic profession, which represents Medicine's biggest competition. So much so, that there have been articles appearing in medical journals expounding the virtues of why chiropractic care is the world's fastest growing health profession, and that physicians should learn from chiropractors how to handle patients – panic sets in when droves of patients begin to seek non-traditional care.

This next bit of news may shock you; acting courses were being offered to physicians at a university in London, Ontario, Canada. Their purpose was to teach doctors how to be empathetic toward their patients. And for those who cannot be empathetic, you can always act Brilliant!

If the above bit of news shocked you, hang onto your hat – you may find the next tid-bit even more unsettling:

In a very recent research study just published in February, 2005,[25] in the American Medical Journal of Bone and Joint Surgery, the authors concluded that basic musculoskeletal knowledge is essential to the practice of Medicine. What a concept! I totally agree. I feel strongly that all physicians should know that the knee bone is attached to the hip bone, etc. As a matter of fact, I feel that this knowledge is crucial for a doctor. With that in mind, the authors of the study tested the knowledge of basic musculoskeletal principles in a number of medical disciplines in order to ascertain physician training adequacy.

Here are the results:

a. The average score was 56.9%. *(This is an F grade.)*
b. Only 21% scored 73.1%, the recommended passing grade.
c. 79% flunked the test. *(Scary.)*
d. 82% of medical students in their last month of training failed.
e. 100% of these students failed the anatomy section of the test. *(Where is that bottom disc anyway?)*
f. 46% of those who stated that they were very comfort able with performing a patient examination, had an average score of only 66%. *(A comforting thought.)*

And the public is asked to trust that their doctor knows what he is doing?

Considering that musculoskeletal problems are the largest group of complaints (second only to respiratory conditions) that physicians handle, this is a very unsettling thought.

---

[25] Matzkin Elizabeth, et al, "Adequacy of Education in Musculoskeletal Medicine," *Journal of Bone and Joint Surgery*, Feb 2005; 87:310-314.

SLUR CAMPAIGN

In order to eliminate competition, Medicine has embarked on a slur campaign against Chiropractic hoping they can sway public opinion in their own direction. For instance, some time ago, the American Medical Association formed what was then called the Anti-Quackery Committee. Its sole purpose was to discredit the Chiropractic profession in the public eye. It was also the policy of the Association to chastise any physician who referred a patient to a chiropractor. A number of years later, Dr. Chester Wilk and a small group of dedicated chiropractic doctors decided to launch a class action suit against the American Medical Association, the American Hospital Association, and the American College of Radiologists. They won! Similar action has also been seen in Canada.

The Canadian Medical Association, although not publicly stated, frowns on physicians who have any type of rapport with chiropractic doctors. As a matter of fact, the Ontario Medical Association's apparent policy seems to be to harass any Ontario physician who does not tow the party line of the Association. I am referring to the case of Dr. Joseph Kropf, an Ontario physician, who lost his case with the OMA for simply prescribing vitamins and natural products to a patient rather than drugs. Such is the control that medical associations and the pharmaceutical industry have over you, the patient – not a good thing. Do you still believe that this is all done for your good health?

TOO MANY ORGANS

Medicine, it appears, seems to be based on two theories: One is that people have too many organs, and the other is that our bodies lack toxic chemicals. These two theories are responsible for you, the patient, accepting the advice of your physician. The sobering thought here is that we, as the public, have accepted this line of reasoning as the truth. We have been *taught* to think that the reason a person has headaches is because they have a lack of Tylenol or Advil in their system. That low back pain is the result of a Robaxacet deficiency. That heartburn is directly attributable to a shortage of Gaviscon, or Pepcid AC, or Zantac. Also that depression is caused by a "chemical imbalance," and is due to a scarcity of Prozac in the body. This has been carefully contrived and orchestrated by organized medicine and the pharmaceutical industry for one purpose only – profit. It's a brilliant marketing scheme. The terrifying fact is that ordinary people have accepted this marketing plan as health care.

Let's look at this a little closer.

Your spouse has just returned from visiting with the family physician and was diagnosed with XYZ disease or syndrome. The doctor mentions that he happens to have just the right drug for this condition. The doctor also mentions that if he cannot solve this problem then the organ will need to be removed because, for some reason, it is not working. There seems to be no thought given to the *"WHY."* There appears to be no concept and no weight given to the idea that there could be a reason behind this strange malady. We seem to accept this on face value and that is it. No one questions why a certain organ suddenly decided to fail – all by itself. Why would this happen doesn't even cross our conscious thought! Think of this for just a moment;

We tend to equate our bodies to a car, for instance. Parts fail and we seem to be OK with that – just part of having a car. Right? Wrong.

Your automobile is a man-made structure. Your body is not – it is a self-repairing, self-regulating entity. What I'm saying is that organs don't suddenly fail. Have I got your interest yet? Wonderful, let's go on.

Let me illustrate just how bizarre our thinking tends to be. Actually, what is even more bizarre is our acceptance of this type of thinking. In many dealings with my patients, they would often mention that they have depression, Colitis, Asthma, Infertility, or whatever. When I ask them *why* they have it, they are totally stunned. To an average earthling, that is a very bizarre question. But, I am serious. I continue to ask them *why* they think they have their particular condition. A huge silence follows that question. People seem to accept that it is OK to be sick and really don't question the idea that they are sick, or why.

The learned thinking is to accept that there is a drug out there that will solve their condition. I find this a chilling concept, and yet we have learned that this is quite normal thinking. I don't know about you, but I feel it is very frightening to think this way.

I mentioned this concept earlier – the drug industry is on a band wagon to "create" new diseases in order to sell more drug and it seems that most of this fervor is targeting women. I spoke of the "Overactive Bladder Disease" for instance, well now they are trying to create a new disorder for which new drugs can be administered. It is known as "female sexual dysfunction" in order to build markets for drugs among women, despite controversy surrounding the medicalization of sexual problems, said an article in the *British Medical Journal*. Many researchers believe that portraying sexual difficulties as a dysfunction will encourage doctors to prescribe drugs that change sexual function, when attention should be paid to other aspects of a woman's life. It's also likely to make women think they have a malfunction when they do not. But perhaps the greatest concern is the ever-narrowing definitions of "normal" that help turn the complaints of the healthy into the conditions of the sick, the study warned. Scary stuff.[26]

Get a load of this: I picked up a copy of *USA Today* recently, and it contained a May, 2005, insert from the American Gastroenterological Association (AGA) entitled, "Digestive Insight." The focus was heartburn.

There were only two suggestions the AGA made for those suffering from Heartburn: a. Change your diet; b. Make your way to the drugstore. Imagine that!

Here is what they said: "Often, diet modifications aren't enough, or they *take too much effort*." – So, you should live on drugs. Wonderful!

But, the key to the article was the fact that they made simple heartburn into a disease. Yes. It is now called "GERD" or, "Gastro-esophageal Reflux Disease."[27] And, you guessed it, there are a myriad of comforting drugs out there which they can sell you – because you now have a disease.

---

[26] Moynihan Ray; "The making of a disease: female sexual dysfunction," *BMJ*, January 4, 2003, Vol 326, 45-47.

[27] Digestive Insight, The American Gastroenterological Association, May 2005.

Isn't it a wonderful service they are providing for us gullible Earthlings? The real frightening thing is that there is a whole section in this insert which deals with pediatric GERD – yes, babies are being targeted – Wonderful!

That same paper also contained another insert, this one from the "Asthma and Allergy Foundation of America" – four pages of drug info and their benefits – nothing about alternative ways of dealing with these problems. Why?

Simple – there is no profit in it.

FEAR

Medicine seems to work on the framework of fear. The fear that is most prevalent is the fear of loss. For example, someone may be thinking that if they don't do exactly what the doctor tells them to do they will lose something; a limb, an arm, an organ, your spouse's life, your child's life and perhaps your own. We then become very motivated to listen to the doctor. We tend to look at the family doctor in terms of salvation because he is going to save us from our fate. Our fate is the loss of a limb, a life, or whatever. Medicine, as a practice, has operated on that basis for years. The doctor has always been regarded more highly than anyone else in society simply because they have specialized knowledge that everyone else doesn't.

This situation has been very manipulative. If a physician really wanted to push this point of power, he would simply say to a patient (and see if I am correct about this), "If you don't do this or if you go there and don't take my advice, I will stop being your doctor." Talk about fear. Talk about coercion. Talk about extortion. The difficulty with this concept is that people have actually done very little about it. My feeling is that if you, as a parent, are ever told words to that effect, you should fire your doctor - they are not working in your best interests – that may be a very good thing to do. Maybe people should do this more often. Now, I am not incubating a rebellion here, just the use of common sense.

For years Medicine has always been empowered. This has clearly been seen throughout the ages and is common in all cultures.

One of the biggest fears of organized allopathic medicine has been the loss of power, the loss of public face, and the loss of public stature. In the past, this has been seen as ridicule of any idea that even remotely transgresses the principles of Medicine. Organized medicine even to present day still works on this principle. If there is a profession out there that cannot, or will not kowtow to the influence of modern allopathic medicine, then two things happen. Either that profession is absorbed into mainstream medical thought or, even more prevalent, it is eliminated completely. Refer to the profession of Osteopathy, for example. Here is a profession that was in direct competition with organized medicine and, as a result, was absorbed. Presently, osteopathic doctors perform surgery, prescribe medication, and have almost all but forgotten their own profession and art.

The very real fear of Organized Medicine is the fact that Alternative medicine is coming to the forefront. The American Medical Association in its May, 1998, Journal,[28] reported that North Americans are following a Japanese lead, turning in massive numbers to so-called "alternative medicine." The reason is that people think it works better. Stanford researchers, on the basis of a national study, estimate that Americans made 425 million visits to alternative health care providers in 1990, a figure that exceeded the number of visits to allopathic primary care physicians during the same period by almost 100 million visits. (47 percent of these physicians also reported using alternative therapies themselves, while 23 percent incorporated them into their practice). According to the JAMA article, the two most frequently endorsed benefits are, "I get relief for my symptoms, reducing the pain or discomfort," or "the treatment works better for my particular health problem than standard medicine." According to the study author, these responses were unexpected and he suggests that its perceived efficacy is the most influential or salient factor in a patient's decision to use alternative health care.[29] So what's the catch?

Drugs kill. Vitamins, amino acids, herbs, and minerals are not only safe, easy to obtain, and far less expensive than prescription drugs, but they seem to promote health and make many pharmaceuticals

---

[28] Why Patients Use Alternative Medicine, JAMA, May 20, 1998,. 1548-1553.
[29] Life Without Limits, The Asthma and Allergy Foundation of America, May 2005.

unnecessary. The clinical experience of medical doctor Robert C. Atkins in his book *Vita-Nutrient Solution* confirms the Stanford survey. Many vitamins, minerals, herbs, amino acids and various other non-toxic "vital" substances are more therapeutically effective than dangerous drug counterparts!

To make this real for you, allow me to give you Comparative Causes of Death Annual Averages in the U.S.:[30]

Adverse Drug Reactions	100,000 - 280,000
Automobile Accidents	41,325
Food Contamination	9,100
Boating Accidents	2,064
Household Cleaners	74
Acute Pesticide Poisoning	12
All Vitamins	0
Amino Acids	0
Herbal Products	0

We now know why the pharmaceutical industry feels compelled to spend massive amounts of money on drug advertising aimed at our children – the future survival of two industries is at stake: funeral parlors and pharmaceuticals! There you have it!

Take heart, however, the tide is beginning to swing the other way – people are beginning to realize that drugs are not health care. There are more and more articles appearing in major newspapers across North America: The Toronto Star did a wonderful six part series on the most common drugs and their problems, in December of 2004. In April ,2004, Reporter Alan Young wrote a wonderfully sarcastic article on Big Pharma in the Toronto Star: "Big Pharma is in the business of sickness and it's in their best interest to maintain a horde of sick people as consumers. When medicine is driven by business objectives, the healing perspective gets skewed. For example, painfully shy people are

---

[30] Source Data from American Association of Poison Control Centers, National Center for Health Statistics, Journal of the American Medical Association, Centers for Disease Control, March of Dimes, Consumer Product Safety Commission, FDA Reports.

[31] Young Alan, Healing Practices Corrupted by Big Pharma, Toronto Star, April 11, 2004.

no longer simple introverts, but suffer 'social anxiety disorder.' Conveniently, Zoloft is available to cast out the demons of shyness."[31] Right!

So you see, things are beginning to change – but it starts with you! Are you willing to help?

And I just have to add this: while on vacation on Hilton Head Island, I picked up the July, 2005, issue of *Free Wheelin'*,[32] an RV publication. Did you know that in 1904, just 100 years ago, 90 percent of all U.S physicians had no college education? That two of the leading causes of death were Stroke and Heart Disease? (in 100 years, we haven't budged an inch) That 95 percent of all births took place at home?

* * *

And the last word…

As a retired physician, I can honestly say that unless you are in a serious accident, your best chance of living to a ripe old age is to avoid doctors and hospitals and learn nutrition, herbal medicine and other forms of natural medicine. Almost all drugs are toxic and are designed only to treat symptoms and not to cure anyone. Vaccines are highly dangerous, have never been adequately studied or proven to be effective, and have a poor risk/reward ratio. Most surgery is unnecessary and most textbooks of medicine are inaccurate and deceptive. Almost every disease is said to be idiopathic (without known cause) or genetic – although this is untrue. In short, our mainstream medical system is hopelessly inept and/or corrupt. The treatment of cancer and degenerative diseases is a national scandal. The sooner you learn this, the better off you will be.

-A. Greenberg, M.D.

Dear Dr. Ressel,

Every parent wants the best for their children and as the parents of five children, aged two to eight years, meeting this challenge is no small feat.

Our children were born either in a family birth centre or in our own home with the assistance of midwives. For years now we've

<hr>

[32] *Free Wheelin'*, Southeastern Publishing, July 2005, Acworth GA.

eaten organically grown and processed foods whenever possible. So chiropractic was a welcome alternative to traditional medical practises, which tend to rely on prescription drugs.

Chiropractic has become part of our proactive approach to Wellness. Our children are learning to listen to their bodies and to use their bodies' natural ability to cope with illness without the use of drugs. Chiropractic in an integral part of our healthy lifestyle.

-Doreen Nicoll and Ed Killen

3. Chiropractic
Handmade Health Care

Chiropractic, as you probably know, has been scoffed at in the media, ridiculed, criticized as being unscientific, and generally harassed because it is different, and based on totally different healing principles than allopathic Medicine. For years traditional Medicine has attempted to discredit the profession of Chiropractic as being cultist, unscientific, etc. Nothing could be further from the truth. The reason is quite simple. Chiropractic is competition. Medicine fears our profession because of its increasing popularity, public dislike of drugs, fear of drug side-effects, and the fact that it is based on healing principles which appeal to people; they are honest, logical, scientific, and make sense to the average person.

To put the shoe on the other foot, Professor David Eddy of North Carolina was quoted in a recent research paper entitled, "Where is the Wisdom – The Poverty of Medical Evidence,"[33] where he stated that only 15 percent of medicine is based on solid science. The rest is based on conjecture, opinion, whims and 'flights of fancy.' Only approximately one percent of medical research has any credibility and is based on scientific thought." There you have it!

Many people ask why the professions of Chiropractic and Medicine do not get along. My answer is actually very simple. Both professions are diametrically opposed when approaching an individuals' health. As I mentioned earlier, Medicine is essentially "crisis control" and seems to work in "opposites." Let me illustrate. If you have high blood pressure, they will give you a drug to lower it. If your pressure is too low they will raise it. If your heart is beating quickly, they will slow it down. If it is beating too slowly, they will increase it. If your stomach is producing too much acid, your physician will give you a drug to lower it. If it is not producing enough, he will give you something else to stimulate acid production. Yes, the whole medical system seems to be based on creating the opposite effect. And on it goes *ad nauseum*.

---

[33] Smith, R., "Where is The Wisdom—the Poverty of Medical Evidence," *British Medical Journal*, Oct. 5, 1991:303(6806):798-9.

No one ever asks 'WHY' this would be occurring in your body. Think about this for a moment; why would your body not produce enough stomach acid, for example? Interesting question isn't it?

PRINCIPLES OF HEALTH

OK ... you now realize that Medicine works in creating the opposite effect in the Body. Chiropractic, on the other hand, is very different. It is based on four very important and profound principles. In a nutshell, they are:

1. SELF-HEALING

Your body is a self-healing, self-regulating organism. It is designed to heal itself and regulate all its own functions. Many patients are surprised when I mention that once a month, they get a brand new liver. Liver cells die and you get new ones approximately every 24 days. What an amazing concept! The next time you are at a party you can amaze your neighbors with this fact. Listen to this; every four months, all your red blood cells are replaced, like clockwork, for the rest of your life! What an awesome thought!

When you go home in the evening and change your clothes as you get ready for bed, you literally shed millions of skin cells in the process. They float in the air and drop onto your carpet. Did you know that 98 percent of all the dust in your house is made up of dead skin cells? You actually vacuum up yourself when you clean the house. This sounds gross, doesn't it? But it is very true. So, the point I am making is that your body is designed to repair and heal itself. In order for it to do that, however, it must follow a very exact program that is set into motion almost from the time you are conceived. I always have fun with my patients when I am doing my consultations because I always ask them "I want to know why you, Betty, are not following your program. Think about this for a moment – what is preventing your body from doing what it is designed and programmed to do?"

Ponder this for a moment: when you are not well, your body is not following your program. Sounds simple and logical, doesn't it? And yet for most people this is a very foreign thought – you have been trained to learn that drugs are the answer to your health quest! The alarming thought is that as adults, you still think this way! ... And the most damaging aspect of this is that you pass these bizarre principles of drugs and health onto your children.

Not OK!

2. COMPUTER CONTROL

The second principle is even more interesting. It is based on the fact that the nervous system is the master controller of the body. It is like a computer control system that runs you! It runs and executes your program. As long as your nervous system is able to communicate effectively with every cell, tissue, every nook and cranny of you, you then should have the very best health you have ever had in your life. We simply call this normal. It's what being healthy is all about!

3. INTERFERENCE

Here is where this gets really cool: if your nervous system is not able to communicate with every tissue, cell, and nook and cranny of you, for whatever reason, your body will not be able to do what it is programmed and designed to do. In other words, you will not be *able* to follow or execute your own program. Your body will start to do its own "thing." We call this Malfunction ... And Malfunction can take many different forms: I'll discuss these in detail in a page or two.

4. COMMUNICATION BREAK

My responsibility as a Doctor of Chiropractic is to simply restore Law & Order. To locate areas in your spine where there is a break in this communication. Such a break interferes with your normal nervous system function – an area of your spine where the nerve signal is being interrupted or interfered with. Chiropractors call these areas of interference *vertebral subluxations*. Our mission is simple: correct any vertebral subluxations so that normal nerve function is restored. This will make the nervous system able to communicate and control body functions once again – health is the result!

Let's look at this process in light of a child who has conditions that I see quite often: Crohn's disease, Ulcerative colitis, stomach ulcers, Asthma, bed-wetting, Colic, ear infections, "growing pains," A.D.H.D. (Attention Deficit Hyperactivity Disorder), or any other myriad of illnesses for which parents bring their children to our Centre or any other wellness chiropractor.

NEUROLOGY FOR DUMMIES

You need to understand that your brain controls you – totally. It controls the function of every organ, cell and tissue; your brain and nervous system control every part of your being. Your nervous system is comparable to a Super Computer that runs the whole show. In order for your brain to communicate effectively with your body, however, there must be a connection between the brain and the body. That connection is called the spinal cord – part of your nervous system. For those of you, who are not very clinically oriented, think of the spinal cord as a telephone cable containing millions of tiny "wires," called nerves. They originate in your brain and travel along your spinal cord to different parts of your body; the longest nerve in your body being the sciatic nerve – it can be up to seven feet long. That's a lot of nerve! The function of these nerves is to transmit information and messages between your brain and your body so that you can execute your program and maintain normal function and health. Isn't that amazing?

The above message transmission is referred to as *Synaptic Transmission*. The nerve has to fire information across a tiny space – a synapse, between the nerve and what is called, the end organ. This system relies on the release of neurotransmitter chemicals to affect message transmission. Synaptic transmission is the conventional thought when people envision a "pinched nerve."

Very recent evidence, however, points to a system that utilizes non-synaptic transmission to cause an effect on body function. This research is brand new and deals with the idea of "wave propagation" and tone. It was discovered that messages sent by the nervous system could travel through wave amplification centers and affect other, neighboring centers through resonance. Sounds complicated? Not really. Imagine holding a tuning fork that is vibrating in the proximity of one that is not. You'll note that the vibration of one will start to affect the other. Thus, information is transmitted throughout the body by non-synaptic means.

To complicate matters even more, recent evidence by Sturm, points to a "chaotic construct" and individual cell neuronal synchronization – cell message centers – let's leave it at that for the time being.

The bottom line is that if the nervous system is allowed to function normally and transmit information from the brain to the body and from the body to the brain with nothing interfering in this process, then you should have the best health you've ever had. That is simply called normal.

Imagine, however, taking a knife and cutting the spinal cord in half between the neck and the shoulders. How many of you suspect that this would not be a good thing to do? You are right. We have just caused a serious breach in communication between the brain and the rest of you. It would mean instant death.

MALFUNCTION

If on the other hand, we caused a small interference in the spinal cord making only part of your nervous system inoperative, the rest transmitting information fairly normally, your body would then not function normally. In other words, your body would no longer be able to follow the program. It would malfunction.

Let's look at this closer. Consider, for example, driving your brand new Lincoln. Instead of having it running on eight cylinders, as it should, it is now only running on five. The dashboard warning bells, whistles and lights are all on, there is smoke appearing in the back of the vehicle and at every stoplight it stalls. But generally, it is still driveable. This would be a good example of malfunction.

Your body is similar. It can still function to a degree but it would not be what we call good health. I call this survival or just simply getting by. It is not OK. Yet, to many of us this seems to be the normal operating state for a human being. We even *expect* this state of affairs when we "get older," and over our lifetime we surround ourselves with things we are no longer able to do. It soon becomes a wall so high we are unable to see over it. That is not health.

What would be examples of malfunction in the body? Let's see … stiffness of movement (especially in the morning), numbness and tingling in the hands or feet, chronic cough, diarrhea, constipation, wheezing, dribbling in your underwear when you cough or sneeze (yes, the DEPENDS people love you!), ear infections, etc. There are thousands of examples of malfunction.

While I'm on this topic, allow me to say a word on the use of "Depends" or "Attends." In order to chase the prescription god, Medicine must first be able to diagnose your condition. This is very important because once diagnosed, a physician can now write you a prescription.

So, the simple problem of bladder incontinence affecting millions of people has been transformed into a "disease" so that a diagnosis can now be made and a drug can now be prescribed. Yes, this is now called "Overactive Bladder Disease." Have you heard of it? I'll bet you have. Listen up, how bizarre is that concept? Your bladder decided to dribble all by itself? Without your permission? Who is in charge anyway?

DISEASE

If some part of the body is not functioning normally (i.e. malfunctioning) and is allowed to remain in such a state, what do you think would happen given time? The part of your body that is not functioning will start to breakdown and become sick. We call this next step *disease*. Look at this further: When we take the word "disease" and analyze it closely, it is really made up of two separate words – *dis* and *ease*. *Dis* is a Latin derivative meaning "not" and "ease" means "not comfortable." *Dis-ease* then means that your body is not comfortable, not at ease. Medicine took out the hyphen and created this new word called "disease" – something to be feared!

Once we have disease we then give it labels, which we can pick out of thousands of different names, such as Asthma, Colitis, Pneumonia, Bronchitis, Meningitis, etc. This is done because for that name there is—you guessed it, a drug to deal with that particular disease. What a concept!

SYMPTOMS

Consider this scenario for a moment. When you reach a point where your body has had enough, and it can no longer handle this disease "thing," it will actually talk to you in a language you can readily understand. We call that language "symptoms." Very often, your body will scream and we call that symptom *pain*. And, as you know, there are all types of different symptoms. There is pain, there is heartburn, difficult breathing, itching of the skin, watering of the eyes, sputtering, coughing, chest pain, arm pain, numbness, constipation, diarrhea, gas, bloating, bladder incontinence, neck pain, back pain, headaches, etc. There are literally thousands of symptoms. And by now you've guessed there is a drug to deal with every one of those symptoms. Isn't that wonderful? Isn't it a terrific service the drug industry is providing for us? But the really amazing thing is that we accept this as health care. Nothing could be further from the truth.

Let's look at this a little bit further. Let's go back to the child who is sitting in front of me at our Centre and has some of the conditions I have just mentioned. What if I took some miracle drugs, sang some songs, danced, did some magic, sprinkled stardust in this child's eyes, did voodoo, and magically I was able to get rid of their symptoms. This child would now feel terrific. Look Ma, no symptoms! Aha! Would this patient now be healthy? Think about this. Would he/she be healthy?

Absolutely not! What did I just do? Did I correct the problem that caused his body not to function normally, or did I merely get rid of his symptoms? Good question. I simply got rid of his symptoms. That's all I have done. The problem is still present. But this child feels terrific – even though his body is not functioning normally.

Now, you need to think of this from a different perspective. The symptoms that an individual experiences can be likened to an alarm system. Your body possesses its very own alarm system to let you know if you can handle what it is going on inside you. It is similar to having a fire break out in your living room. The alarm system would go off in the house. In that instance, you have a choice – either put out the fire or turn off the alarm system. Guess what most people do? Do you think they search for the cause of the problem and put out the fire, or do they look for a quick fix and turn off the alarm system – the symptoms? You're right! I would estimate that 98 percent of Earthlings are thrilled to just turn off the alarm system, living in happy oblivion until their body finally says at some point "no you don't, I have had enough, this is it, I quit." I mean, if your body were to wear out, where would you live?

The medical/pharmaceutical cartel, as mentioned earlier, is making billions of dollars on this type of thinking. As a matter of fact, they propagate this type of reality because it is very profitable. The more symptoms we deal with, the wealthier the drug industry gets because we are not looking after the problem, which means things will fail down the road and get worse. When this occurs, we will be dependent on drugs to sustain what is left of life. That is our health care system in North America. By now you are either agreeing with me or you are convinced that I'm insane – there is no middle ground!

RECOVERY

Our approach, as chiropractors, is totally different. Instead of putting out the alarm system, let's see if we can correct the interference that caused the nervous system not to function normally in the first place. Would you agree this approach makes more sense? As I mentioned earlier, we call this interference a "vertebral subluxation" – a "misalignment" of one of the vertebrae of the spine that interferes in the manner with which the nervous system transmits information. When a subluxation is in the process of being corrected, you soon notice that symptoms begin to subside and disappear. This does not mean the patient is healthy or the problem is corrected, it just means that the body is more able to handle it on its own. This is a very important distinction. Another positive result is that the malfunction the body has been experiencing starts to subside. In other words, things start to function the way they were actually designed. You are beginning to follow the program again and the disease process actually starts to reverse itself. The pathology begins to heal and you start on the road to recovery. This is very important.

Let me illustrate this point using an analogy I use quite often with my patients: You are standing on a hill in the winter and I hand you a snowball. You fumble it, drop it, and we are chasing it down the hill. Near the bottom, guess what happens to the size of this snowball? You are right, it is huge – we have an avalanche!

At this point, we only have two things that must be accomplished: One, we need to stop the snowball from rolling down the hill further, and two, dig our heels in, shoulder this snowball, and start to roll it back to the top of the hill. In other words, reverse the damage, the pathophysiology, and the pathology. The rest of it, we have all been plagued with *ad nauseum*, such as exercise, vitamins, supplements, diet, nutrition, etc., can be viewed as window dressing. Without these two most important points, the rest of the plethora of self-help that is available to the public will not be effective. Period.

It is because of these profound principles that Chiropractic has set itself apart from allopathic Medicine. Many patients ask me "Why don't chiropractors and physicians get together?" I do not honestly know how to answer that question because the two professions are so vastly different; like oil and water, and I can never see them mixing together successfully. The principles of health and life are so vastly different between both of them.

VERTEBRAL SUBLUXATION

I would like to expand on those strange words I used earlier – the vertebral subluxation. In simple terms, it is a misalignment of the spinal vertebrae. These vertebral subluxations are most often painless but do cause interference in the manner in which your nervous system transmits information all over your body. Deepak Chopra M.D. once stated, "The mysterious breakdowns in the body's intelligence … may be traceable to a single distortion, a wrong detour …"

A distortion in the function and alignment of your spine will cause your body to malfunction and this will eventually produce a state of disease. Chiropractors have spent years studying how to locate and correct subluxations of the spine, thereby allowing your nervous system to function normally. This eventually reconnects you to the innate intelligence that runs your body – all without drugs or surgery. What an amazing discovery! Let me give you some examples of how truly amazing it is.

Infant Apnea—A case of Medical Mayhem and Ignorance

A young father came to my clinic recently looking haggard and emotionally exhausted. He had just returned from vacation with his wife but did not radiate the typical picture of a good holiday. He informed me that his wife gave birth to their first child, Breanna, just a week ago and the baby stopped breathing one hour and twenty minutes after delivery. An obstetrician at a local hospital delivered the baby. The delivery was induced and the mother was given an epidural block (more on epidurals in a later chapter). An APGAR numerical score of one to ten is given to an infant at birth, and five minutes after, to determine the stress of delivery on the baby. APGAR stands for Activity, Pulse, Grimace (crying ability), Appearance of the skin, and Respiration. A perfect score would be 10.

In young Breanna's case, the APGAR score was noted to be 6 at birth, and 8 at 5 minutes. For the average human, this is a normal uncomplicated delivery. Little Breanna was resuscitated and subjected to a variety of tests like CT SCAN, EEGs, etc. The results were inconclusive. No reason for cessation of breathing was found. She was transferred to a neonatal unit at a university teaching hospital and was placed under the care of a pediatric neurologist. There, she baffled the best of the best and went into respiratory arrest every twenty minutes. In the true sense of allopathic lunacy, she was placed on a course of antibiotic therapy for a few days, then prescribed phenobarbitol for the possibility of seizures, as well as vitamins. Brilliant!

She was released from the hospital and sent home with a twenty-four hour breathing monitor. This device monitored her breathing patterns and went off every twenty minutes over the course of the next few weeks. I do not need to tell you the mental and emotional state of the parents. As a matter of fact, the parents were told to pick up their child from her crib and shake her like a clock so that she would literally start ticking.

I saw Breanna at two and half weeks of age, "a beautiful young child." The mother mentioned that forceps were not used but my visual inspection and examination of the head indicated otherwise. There was considerable molding and asymmetry of the head. The neurological signs seemed to be within normal limits and Breanna would feed from her mother's breast with little difficulty. When I checked for vertebral subluxations, I found problems at the first and second vertebrae in the spine, which affect the manner in which the spinal cord transmits information.

That particular area of the spine deals with the respiratory centers, which seemed to be suppressed. After two months of care, Breanna's breathing monitor had disappeared and she was able to breathe very happily on her own. What never ceases to amaze me is how the current medical system simply cannot find a correlation between traumatic birth (which I will talk about in detail later) and its affect on the respiratory centers. A second quarter chiropractic student could have figured this out. All in all, dealing with little Breanna and her family has been a pleasure. It is overwhelming to see the power of innate.

Cyclic Vomiting Syndrome

Another case that comes to mind is of a ten year-old girl named Alison, who came to the clinic recently with a chronic stomach problem. She was diagnosed with Cyclic Vomiting Syndrome (CVS). I doubt that anyone reading this book would have heard of this condition. I certainly never have and I deal with pediatrics almost exclusively. Apparently, there are only a handful of people across Canada and the rest of the world who have this strange disease – and she was one of the lucky ones. As a matter of fact, there is a town northwest of Toronto that has a world CVS support group where parents fly in from all parts of North America to talk about their children's condition and learn how to cope with it—and deal with it. I feel that coping and dealing with a condition is distasteful and it runs against everything I have ever learned about health care. Why would you want to cope and deal with something when you can actually have the possibility of wiping it out? This girl's symptoms were absolutely bizarre – she would start to retch and vomit for no apparent reason to the point where she would actually vomit blood. The vomiting was severe and debilitating.

When I first met Alison, I had to ask myself why a beautiful ten-year old girl would be afflicted with such a condition. There must be a reason. This was not a normal state of affairs. Following my intuition and training, I decided to check the state and function of her nervous system. I found she had a vertebral subluxation in her spine that affected the part of her nervous system which controlled her stomach function. After the subluxation was corrected, the vomiting stopped and has not come back since. The parents and the child were thrilled, but at the same time a little upset that they could no longer belong to the support group because of their child's recovery. The support group had become a big part of their social life. The recovery of the daughter had now created a whole different set of social circumstances. They now had to find a different circle of friends.

Although you might laugh and find this bizarre, many patients I meet have had a problem for a number of years and consider their problem to be their pet gorilla, which they feed, stroke, fondle, and hang on to. If you think what I am saying is fanatical, then just think of the friends you have with a health condition and how they take care of it. In many cases, just having a health problem becomes their whole life. Think of your aunt Betty who loves to talk about her bowels! We are very strange creatures, we human beings.

CAUSES OF SUBLUXATIONS

You may be thinking at this point, "Where do subluxations come from?" How do you get these things? Do you find them in your cereal, do you find them in your soup, and do they descend upon you from the heavens? No, most of them are caused by trauma, and a percentage is caused by stress (emotional and even chemical.) The most common cause of vertebral subluxations (85 percent) is actually caused by the birth and delivery process. In other words, the way you were brought into the world. Birth. Yes! Let me ask you this: How many of you have had this experience? See my drift? In other words, the stress and pressure of actually being squeezed through a little tiny 10 centimeter canal and someone grabbing your head and twisting it and pulling you out.

There are also many other causes of vertebral subluxations such as car accidents, old habits, poor posture, sport injuries. The list is endless. Birth, however, is number one. It is for this reason that many chiropractors put a great amount of emphasis on children and infants. As a matter of fact, our Centre was probably one of the few in North America that was totally devoted to children. I must add that although I am no longer in active practice, my mission is still the same: To help as many people in my lifetime as I can – especially children! I now teach other doctors how to do it through my Practice Evolution Program.

I feel it is imperative for parents to have children checked at an early age to ensure optimal health and development for life. As a society, it should be our highest calling.

* * *

My son, James, was born at 25 weeks gestation and weighed one pound six ounces. He is the sole survivor of triplets. Little did I know what lay ahead of me, with the problems I would have with this little guy for the next few years.

James was in the hospital for four and a half months. During this time he was incubated and was tube fed, which meant he was on oxygen and had problems with his lungs. Chronic Lung Disease, three blood transfusions, apnea problems (stopped breathing) along with having to be suctioned through his nose and throat. He had to have emergency surgery for a bilateral inguinal hernia problem and was on many medications (including antibiotics).

After James' tubes were removed and he was breathing room air without the help of an oxygen tank for many days at a time, it was then time to try to breast feed him. This was very unsuccessful since James had not learned what we would call the "sucking reflex" which most people feel is automatic and natural. James could not latch onto my breast very well, and when he did, he didn't know when to suck, breathe and when to swallow and in what order. He repeatedly turned blue and would lose weight since it was so much work for him. Since James could not suck, I had to make the hole in the nipples of his bottle larger. For James it was an ongoing battle until he finally learned how to suck through a straw at age four.

*Gaining weight was and still is an ongoing concern since he was diagnosed with "**failure to thrive**" problem he had "Gastroesophageal Reflux Disease," where he would projectile vomit all the time every-day and have continuous ear infections. Along with that he had eating problems. Every day five to six times a day we would sit in the high chair and try to eat a small meal. James would be okay with food that was pureed but it had to be from the baby food jar, not something I would make because it couldn't have one bit of chunk in it or he would throw up and gag from the texture. At nine months of age he decided that he wasn't going to have that nipple in his mouth, so since then he has been drinking from a cup. James's first chunky food with texture was an Arrowroot cookie that he would put in his mouth and drool all over until it would* *dissolve in his mouth. This was the turning point for him. He only started eating pasta when he was over three years old and rice at four. Although choosing foods for James to eat is still frustrating, as he now became picky of what he eats. He likes to stick to yoghurt, custard, pudding, cereals (finger type ones), and of course, cookies.*

As for failure to thrive, since James had so many problems with eating, and having ongoing sicknesses like ear infections and colds, naturally it would affect his growth and appetite. James ear infections would come back within a few weeks to one month, after being on repeated antibiotics and many kinds. Every month I'd take him to get weighed at the doctor's office, and we would see a specialist for preemie babies. We would also see an occupational therapist, nutritionist and pediatrician, to name a few. I would wait anxiously every month to get James weighed, hoping for some kind of weight gain, but the report would usually be anywhere between no weight gain and six ounces weight gain. Nothing to get excited about. At one time I was adding tablespoons of vegetable oil in his cereal to add calories. James was always below average. As time went on, James went through a series of assessments where he was "labeled" DEVELOPMENTALLY DELAYED. He didn't walk until he was twenty-six months old. James has always been at least one and a half years behind the average child at his age. Now James gets a lot of help with teacher from his day care.

As a parent dealing with all of James' problems, and by going to these specialists, which I felt was time-consuming, I discovered their therapies were only temporary band-aid fixes. As a frustrated parent I still was looking for help when I turned to an alternative, that only lack of knowledge has stopped me from getting to it sooner. It is then that I met Dr. Ressel. Of course, I'm always a skeptic when it comes to things I've never heard before, and always thinking that it's some kind of scam.

I gave it a chance and I had to try it out for myself (for James). James is now four and a half years old and 25 pounds. Dr. Ressel's method and philosophy just makes sense – it's that plain and simple. After James began his intense of chiropractic care, he grew, literally two inches in sixteen days and gained one pound in a month. Not only has he been eating like crazy and "new food," he is finally using the toilet (no more diapers), his language skills have improved greatly in such a short period of time, and there haven't been any ear infections to speak about. You wouldn't believe it! Although I don't advise totally ruling out your family doctor, I believe you would only have to see them less when you have chiropractic care. I'm only sorry that media, government, and the health care systems aren't educated   in the field of chiropractic about how important it is, and the benefits that it brings.

-Michelle Gipp

I was introduced to chiropractic care about a year and a half ago through a health and wellness seminar offered in a nearby city. I came upon this type of health care quite by accident and although I didn't seek chiropractic adjustments for a particular symptom or illness, I did suffer from weekly headaches, occasional lower backaches and tension in my neck and shoulder area.

I am a Type 1 diabetic, and due to my illness, am quite familiar with doctors and specialists. Since I was new to chiropractic I tried to stay neutral until I could experience more of its results. However, I was impressed immediately with the type of care I received from Dr. Ressel and his staff. Too many times in traditional medical situations I experienced, I felt like a number or felt that no one was really listening to me. Diagnosis or opinions were almost anticipated before hearing all of the facts, and prescriptions for everything were handed out readily.

From my first visit to my most recent adjustment, I have never been ignored, interrupted or 'assembly-line' diagnosed by Dr. Ressel or his associates. My neutral position quickly changed after noticing that any medical problems I discussed with Dr. Ressel were corrected through chiropractic adjustments or other nonmedicinal suggestions. I rarely get headaches now and my backaches have decreased. If they do occur, I rarely have to reach for pain medication. In the past, my shopping list regularly included acetaminophen, muscle relaxants, and heartburn medications.

I keep referring to health and well-being when I talk about chiro-practic care, but I actually have an overall feeling of well-being since receiving chiropractic care. I am more aware of my body's signals and reactions than ever before. I guess that is why they say subluxations cause an interference, because as these subluxations are corrected these interferences disappear and I no longer feel like the "kinked garden hose" operating only at half capacity.

Chiropractic care has completely changed my way of thinking about my health. Traditional medicine practices seem to be determined to provide quick fixes to get rid of symptoms, but don't seem as dedi-cated to finding the underlying cause of the symptoms. I don't believe enough emphasis is put on finding out why an illness or symptom is experi-enced. Unfortunately, too many people are given quick fixes with disastrous consequences.

The chiropractic philosophy of health and wellness has taught me to be more in charge of my health, to ask more questions, and to demand a higher level of care in any treatment I pursue. Dr. Ressel is committed to ensuring that his patients are well informed and are able to make knowledgeable decisions.

I look forward to my chiropractic care and the continued bene-fits they provide to my health. I am so convinced of these benefits that I will always discuss any medical problems with my chiropractor before another health practitioner and I am always confident that he is listen-ing and will provide the best possible care that he is able to provide.

-Cindy Whitehead

4. Innate Intelligence

It has been coined the 'Wisdom of the Body" by some, "Nature" by others, and "The Force" by George Lucas, producer of Star Wars. Chiropractors refer to this "thing" as **Innate Intelligence** and it simply refers to your body's own organization ability and its ability to self-heal, self-regulate and self-adapt. Deepak Chopra said it best when he mentioned that *"Intelligence is present everywhere in our bodies ... our own intelligence is far superior to any we can try to substitute from the outside."* I am sure that most of you will understand this concept, but for those who have difficulty we'll start off at the very beginning – before you were actually you.

Consider an example of an egg traveling down the Fallopian tubes, which is part of the monthly cycle which every woman experiences. When a woman ovulates, the egg travels down one Fallopian tube one month and then the other tube the next month, in order to give one or the other a break. Who decides how this occurs? Is there an internal clock? Scientists have been trying to figure out what starts this process and, so far, no one has even come close. This is an example of the intelligence of the body.

Let's look at this further. Can you imagine for a moment that there is no egg going down either Fallopian tube, but there are sperm cells in the area – millions of them. Those sperm cells have one mission—to find and unite with an egg. That is their only goal. If there is no egg going down, then the sperm cells are unable to fulfill their mission and they will swim haphazardly in every direction possibly for twenty-four hours, at which time they die. Let me ask you this. How do they know that there is no egg on the way down the Fallopian tube for them to join up with? Is there a beacon at the end of the tunnel telling them that this is a false alarm? Think about this for a moment. How do they know?

I can give you another example. Let's suppose that there is an egg moving down the Fallopian tube and there are the same sperm cells in the area. As I mentioned, it is their mission to unite with the egg. In this case, you will notice that every single sperm, millions of them, will swim directly towards the egg. You will not find one of them swimming in the wrong direction. Let me ask you again. How do they know there is an egg coming down the Fallopian tube and in which tube the egg is descending?

This is what we call *Innate Intelligence*. You are thinking – Right.

There is an intelligence that scientists have simply not been able to explain that governs how our bodies actually function. Now, we may be able to take that process and reduce it down to its chemical components, but the question will still remain. What initiates and what drives the process? What "thing" makes your body work?

Once the egg is fertilized, it then starts to divide, and by the way, only one sperm can fertilize the egg. Once this occurs, is there a gate that shuts and keeps the rest of the million sperm out? Again, we have been able to explain this on a chemical level, but we have not been able to explain the forces involved that actually initiate the process. We simply have no idea. Let me repeat that. With all the technology available, we have no idea how this all takes place. This is simply an example of an intelligence running the body.

Let's look at this a little further. Approximately twenty days after conception (if you look at the clump of cells that are multiplying very rapidly), there is order beginning to be created in that clump of cells. The first organ to develop is the brain and nervous system. Can you guess why the brain (the nervous system) is the first organ that gets developed? If your answer is because it is the most important organ in your body, you are correct. The reason your brain is the first organ to develop is because it is the computer that runs the show and decides how the rest of you will develop.

At approximately five weeks, if you look at this fetus, it now has what are called arm buds and leg buds – the beginning of legs and arms, and it has a tail and it has a very distinct spine. You are probably wondering why on earth this fetus has a spine when it is only five weeks old. So let's look at the reasons.

Even as you sit and read this book, your spine has essentially two reasons for being. The first is for support - to keep you upright so you are not a blob of jelly on the floor. That is the reason most people think of and they are absolutely correct. The second reason, which is actually the most important one, and also one that most people can't think of readily, is protection. Your spine, which is made of bone, serves as a protective covering for your spinal cord, which is similar to a telephone cable running inside your spine. As I mentioned earlier, your spinal cord is composed of billions of tiny wires called nerves, which convey messages to the brain from the body and from the brain to the body. It does control the function of every cell and organ in your body. It is your very own internal Internet. Protection is the paramount mission of your spine and all the muscles controlling the movements of your spine. As I mentioned earlier, any interference with the transmission of messages along your nervous system will cause your body to malfunction—not a good thing. Therefore, your spine serves as a protective covering for your delicate nervous system.

One aspect of this I have always found absolutely amazing is the fact that at about this intricate stage of development, you just found out you are pregnant. Yet, all these miraculous activities are taking place inside you and you are not even aware of them. Amazing! There are a number of wonderful photographs done by Leonard Nielsen published in *Life Magazine* in the early 1980s concerning the development of the child in utero. The reason I am mentioning this is that at about twenty weeks or so, he shows a photograph of a fetus moving the thumb in and out of its mouth – in utero. Think about this for a moment. Why would a fetus move the thumb in and out of its mouth? What is it doing?

If your answer is learning to feed, you are correct. The unborn child is actually practicing how to survive; it is practicing how to breast-feed as soon as it is born. Let me ask you this: How does it know how to do this? What course did mom have to take to teach her unborn baby how to do this? None. How does it know how to place the thumb in and out of its mouth? This is what we call an example of Innate Intelligence. A baby instinctively knows exactly what to do. It is the same way with animals such as horses, who know just what to do. A young colt drops to the ground. It stands and runs. It knows what to do with no instruction from its mother. The baby instinctively knows what to do as well. Its own Innate Intelligence guides it through life, and so does ours. Our own intelligence guides us through life on the same level. We just need to be open to listening to it, and be aware that it is there in the first place. Let me give you some examples as to how amazing this really is.

Let's suppose for a moment that you are sitting with your spouse watching TV and the baby is in another room upstairs. You suddenly bolt upright and say to your husband that the baby is crying. Your husband then looks at you as though you have lost your senses, because he has not heard the baby cry. You run up the stairs and lo and behold the baby is crying. My question would be; how did you know? Did you hear the baby? No. Then how did you know? This is an example of instinct. An innate intelligence that whispered in your mind that the baby was crying. I mentioned this earlier, but I generally find that women have this innate instinct "thing" much more finely honed than men do.

If I can even make this clearer, let us pretend that you are sitting at your desk doing your thing at work, and your baby is with the sitter half way across town. You suddenly bolt out of the chair because you have been hit with this overwhelming feeling that things are going badly at home. Now look inside yourself for a moment and acknow-ledge the fact that you know exactly what I am referring to. You drive home and discover that you are correct. The poop has literally hit the fan. Let me ask you. How did you know that something was wrong at home? Your husband would not have had a clue. However, you did. How? This is an example of your innate-intelligence and instinct at work. Amazing isn't it?

There is a force that we have inside us that guides our growth, our development, and our life. Examples of this force are ever present and are in our everyday environment. Look at the life of the monarch butter-fly for example. The monarch butterfly is plentiful in Ontario and the adjacent states, but did you know that this small butterfly flies all the way to Mexico for the winter and then back again. Not only that, but it flies to the same area in Mexico and then back again. How does it know how to do that? Does it use some sort of a GPS guidance system we are unaware of? Is it actually aware of the tremendous distance involved in such travel? I don't think so. I think it is done by instinct. Its own Innate intelligence is guiding its path. The same thing can be said about birds flying south for the winter and covering incredible miles to do it, and yet they come back to the same spot over and over again. We call this Nature or innate intelligence.

My very favorite is the bumblebee. You maybe aware of this, but it never ceases to amaze me. Apparently, according to scientists and computer experts, the bumblebee can't fly. Because of its weight, and ratio of its wings to its weight, the dihedral angle of wind assault, the speed of wing movements and other physical variables, it is mathematically absolutely impossible for a bumblebee to fly. However, bumblebees do not know this and fly anyway, defying all laws of science known to man.

You can see examples of innate intelligence in your own backyard, at least those of you who live in the Northern United States and Canada. Each Autumn, leaves drop from the trees and in the spring they all reappear. How do they know how to do this? We have been able to explain this on a chemical level, but ultimately on a grander scale, it is the work of nature, the work of innate intelligence. No one knows how the process actually begins, and more importantly why. Take an apple for example. When an apple is on the tree, it will never go rotten, however, once it falls down it will rot and worms will attack it. What is the difference between an apple on the ground and an apple on the tree? The difference is life. Chemically and physiologically the two are identical. The difference is that one is alive and one is not.

Did you know, for example, that every second of your life billions of cells in your body are breaking down foods, they are dying, and they are being reborn? Nerves are shooting information all over your very being and your lunch is being turned into muscle cells, heart cells, and skin cells. Damaged tissues are repaired and replaced, germs and cancer cells killed every minute, and the production of your cells and all chemical processes – approximately 150,000 - are being monitored every second. And all this amazing and wondrous activity takes place while you are sleeping, reading, or driving your car. Amazing, is it not? That is called the wisdom of your body – Innate Intelligence.

5. Raising a Drug-free Family

This may sound like a very strange title for a chapter, but you will see very shortly how inundated we really are with medication. You will need to carefully consider whether your day to day actions really agree with a philosophy of not administering drugs to your children. I find that many parents are in denial at this point, because while your intentions are good, you are creating a drug dependent child without even realizing it. Think back to the time when you, as a mother, just gave birth to your baby and the hospital staff placed silver nitrate in your baby's eyes. The medical assumption is that you, as mom, had gonorrhea. Therefore, the baby could go blind if the eyes were not bathed with silver nitrate. I have never understood this procedure, and I find this very insulting to women. Many women don't question this procedure, and what is worse, they are not even aware that this is a routine practice in North American hospitals and birthing centers.

A Vitamin K injection is also given to your baby at birth, just in case there is some sort of problem with clotting of the blood. Why would this happen? Think about this for a moment. Under the perfect guidance of an innate intelligence, your baby was developed from two cells (the egg and the sperm) into forty quadrillion cells in approximately 280 days with all the organs fully formed and functional – a perfect little expression of life. Do you think the power that made that baby would forget the vitamin K? I don't think so! Get a dose of reality! As a matter of fact, recent studies have shown that Vitamin K injections can cause liver failure in infants. Has your doctor informed you of the possible repercussions? No? It's not nice to fool with Mother Nature!

What about the time when your infant child first exhibits a symptom that indicates his/her body is fighting something. (I am very careful not to use the expression, "sick") You may take your baby to your physician with panic in your heart, and the doctor will most likely prescribe some sort of medication to alleviate your child's suffering.

This is all done under the guise of a normal, and rational thing to do. The point I want you to think about carefully, is that this procedure, this "ritual," is being performed by people who love and care for this child the most – the parents. It is these same people who love and care for the baby the most that are convinced that vaccination is very beneficial and so the baby is injected with a foreign gene-altering substance. No mention is made of the potential lethal and long-term consequences of such an action. It's just a routine thing to do – a mindless action.

As this child grows up to be a toddler and perhaps gets an ear infection, the people who love and care for this child consent to antibiotic treatment, as well as Tempra for fever.

When the child is of school age, and has trouble concentrating and sitting still in class, the people who love and care for him the most, take him/her to a physician. Based on the behavioral analysis of the teacher in most cases, the doctor labels the child hyperactive and prescribes Ritalin or another psychotropic drug. With this new chemically-induced behavior the child is rewarded because his calmer behavior pleases the people who love and care for him most.

When this child reaches high school, he may have difficulty with a girlfriend or boyfriend, or have trouble coping with something that upsets him. The people who love and care for him the most will take him to the family physician again, who will prescribe some kind of antidepressant to help him deal with the upset.

And on it goes.

Even worse than the side effects of these drugs, is the message given to our children. From the time they are born, children receive the message that drugs relieve symptoms that make them feel badly, even before their body begins to do something uncomfortable to them. The message is subtle, and slowly their behavior becomes conditioned. This is actually seen as quite normal – and we wonder where the drug problem begins. Do you remember signs stating "Say No to Drugs?" How can we? We have been brainwashed to believe they are good for us.

Let me give you some amazing statistics to prove my point:

* The National Center for Health Statistics reported 14,843 deaths in 1996 as a result of using illegal drugs. For that same period of time, The New England Journal of Medicine reported 16,500 deaths as a result of using anti-inflammatory drugs such as aspirin and ibuprofen – 1,657 more deaths than caused by illegal drugs combined. And that *does not* include deaths caused by legal drugs other than anti-inflammatories.
* The Journal of the American Medical Association reported in February of 2000 that the use of certain psychotropic drugs, like anti-depressants and stimulants, in 2 to 4 year olds *doubled* or even *tripled* between 1991 and 1995
* In 1999, the pharmaceutical industry spent $1.8 billion to advertise prescription drugs, encouraging a projected 21.2 million consumers to "ask their doctors" about a drug they were not using.
* A Merck-Medco Managed Care report found sales of prescription drugs in 1990 to have generated $50 million; by 1998 that figure had risen to $90 million due in part to a 30% increase in the number of users and a 34% increase in days of use per user.
* Forbes magazine in 1999 found that the top 12 pharmaceutical companies generated a profit of $27.3 billion.
* The United States consumes 90% of the world's Ritalin, and production of Ritalin is up 700% since 1990 and nearly 5 million people in the U.S. – mostly children – are on Ritalin.
* Between 1990 and 1996, the number of children in the U.S. using Ritalin grew by 250 percent.

There is a legal, massively funded and astoundingly profitable drug war being waged in this country. The pharmaceutical companies have been educating our society, starting at an increasingly young age, to reach for a drug for every malaise, be it attention deficit, indigestion, headache, depression, shyness, allergies, insomnia, impotence, or virtually anything that may trouble us. At the same time, alternatives have been systematically repressed, ridiculed of legislatively barred from competing. We are creating drug addicts at the preschool level. We are barraged daily with the message that drugs can and should rescue us from every ill and then we cringe and cry "Just say no!" What hypocrisy.

The war on drugs must be waged in our medicine cabinets. Parents must set an example that drugs are not the first option of choice, that many times improved eating habits, exercise, stress-reduction, and other natural approaches will resolve problems with time and commitment – that the quick fix is usually no fix at all. Only when we change our mind-set as a society will we see any true progress in a war on drugs – are you up for the challenge?

Enter Chiropractic. The answer the public is looking for. People like the simplicity, the logic, and the rationale of the chiropractic approach to health care. It makes sense and has tremendous appeal. Nothing is added to the body and nothing is taken out. We simply remove interference to the nervous system so the body can function optimally. I like that; it is clean cut, simple, and honest. One of the other things the public likes about chiropractic and its approach to health care, is that it is *different*. It defies and even stands in the way of allopathic domination.

A good friend of mine in Atlanta, Dr. Eric Plasker, whose practice consists of many children, once told me that the old message used to be, "I am sorry you feel badly, your body is weak and your body needs these drugs to get well." Wellness on the other hand delivers a very profound statement. The new message states, "Your body is strong and has the ability to heal itself. Let's remove the interference so you can get well on your own - you can trust your body."

Let me give you a few examples of how amazing this truly is.

A few years ago I had the pleasure of taking care of a mother and her two boys. Upon one of her visits to the office, I mentioned that it was important that her husband, who was not a patient at the time, be checked for subluxations to make sure his body was functioning normally. I received many excuses. My favorite was that, "We have no time ... my husband is busy ... he leaves early in the morning and does not get home until 8 P.M. Besides that, he has kidney failure and spends three afternoons a week in the hospital on dialysis." Let me ask you, "How many of you would think this would really cramp your lifestyle?

The mention of kidney failure, of course, evoked a typical response from me – thousands of questions. I simply wanted to know more. To make a long story short, the husband of this family did finally come to see me. He was only 31 years old. He mentioned that both kidneys were failing, and he only had ten percent kidney function left. I should mention that we all have two kidneys but can survive with only one. People have two as a backup system in case one fails. In this patient's case however, both were failing – very unusual.

The hospital gave this man approximately two years to live in his present condition. They were searching for a kidney donor in the meantime – for a possible transplant. Unfortunately, he had a rare blood type and his tissue type was difficult to match. A year passed in the search with no results in sight. Finally the hospital mentioned to the family that they should prepare for the eventuality of his untimely demise and make certain the insurance and all other paperwork was in order.

The first question I asked myself when we met was, "Why would two kidneys suddenly decide to fail?" and "Why would they decide to work 90 percent less than normal, on their very own – all by themselves?" I thought it was a good question. I did a complete examination to see if he had any vertebral subluxations affecting the part of his nervous system that controlled kidney function. Guess what I found? If you think it was the "S" word, you are right! Vertebral subluxations! I remember this as if it only happened yesterday. I gave this man an adjustment to correct the subluxation, and then sent him back to the same hospital to retake all the kidney function tests. The next morning the verdict came back that the kidneys were fully functional – 100 percent. There was no longer a kidney problem! You can imagine the reaction of the family. I remember the children running around my clinic crying and laughing. The husband was thrilled. The only tidbit I must add was that his wife was not very happy. I think there were some other plans being made in the background. Although this story had a very happy ending, I lost track of this family when they moved to the west coast.

Another story I would like to share with you is that of little Stewart who was only 18 months old when his mother first brought him to me. Little Stewart was probably the sickest little boy I have ever seen in my life. He had severe Asthma and Bronchitis since the day he was delivered and was on daily antibiotics and "puffers." Although he was only 18 months, he was the unhealthiest child I had ever seen, in spite of all the wonder drugs he was on. A few months after his Subluxations were corrected, Stewart was taken off all medication and today he leads a very healthy, normal life. You would never know he had a health problem if you were to meet him today.

I bet you can relate to this story; a television commercial. This is actually a problem I encountered every day in my practice. The commercial deals with the sale of adult diapers, namely Depends. I am sure you have seen some of these. At the risk of insulting the manufacturer of the diapers (and I am certainly not trying to do that in any way), the television commercials tend to give the impression that it is quite normal to go shopping—and because you are wearing Depend diapers, do your business in your pants at the same time. They allude to the fact that this is actually quite socially acceptable. How many of you would find this bizarre? The manufacturer, however, is attempting to convince you that it is actually normal to loose control of your bladder because now you have diapers to wear should that situation happen. I am most bothered by this type of advertising, because we actually buy into it. I also find it curious that people never ask why adults would suddenly develop bladder problems. We just accept that it is actually quite normal to wet our pants while shopping even though we are only 50 years old. I am suggesting to you that it is *not* OK and is *not* normal.

It is a manufacturer's reality. Once you have bought into that reality, however, they then give it a name. It's called the "Overactive Bladder Disease" I mentioned earlier. I need you to understand this concept because it is very important. For every disease there is a drug, so it is very important that you give the disease a name. It's all part of marketing – and very little to do with health care!

Another story I would like to tell you about is that of an eighteen-month year old girl named Nicole. She was one of three daughters of a young family. From the month of July until February of the following year, she did not sleep more than five minutes in total, if you can believe that. Imagine yourself with a child who does not sleep. On top of that problem, you have to go to work, take care of the house, and look after two other children. If I say to you that these parents were pulling their hair out, I am not far from the truth. They actually coped quite well with this problem by taking turns playing with Nicole all night long. In other words, one parent would play while the other would sleep. The next day they would switch and take turns. I want you to imagine for a moment the stress on the family and the stress on the little girl.

When I checked Nicole, I found that she had a vertebral subluxation at the very top of the neck affecting the manner in which her nervous system functioned. In this way, her nervous system was under constant stress and never able to let its guard down, so to speak, to let the little girl relax and fall asleep easily. I remember that after adjusting this little girl and correcting her subluxation, the parents had to carry her out to the car and she fell asleep before her dad hit the parking lot. I recall the parents calling me later that evening with considerable panic because their child slept for 12 hours without so much as a stir. I would like you to understand that she has been fine ever since. Such is the power of the body's ability to heal and self-regulate – as long as it is allowed to function normally!

While I'm on the topic of raising healthy children, I am really compelled to urge you to keep your children safe – most accidents happen at home especially when the electric kettle is on the fritz. What does your child do? They place their cup of water in the microwave to heat it up so he can make a cup of tea. Not OK! When the timer shuts the microwave oven off, your child will remove his cup from the oven. As he looks into the cup he notes that the water is not boiling. Then, in an instant, the water in the cup "blows up" into his face. His whole face may be blistered and he may have 1st and 2nd degree burns to his face, which may leave scarring. He may also lose partial sight in his eye. While at the hospital, the doctor who is attending will tell you that this is a fairly common occurrence and water (alone) should never be heated in a microwave oven. If water is heated in this manner, something such as a wooden stir stick or a tea bag should be placed in the cup to diffuse the energy.

Here is the scientific "tech" on the matter:

It is caused by a phenomenon known as super heating. It can occur any time water is heated and will particularly occur if the vessel that the water is heated in, is new. What happens is that the water heats faster than the vapor bubbles can form. If the cup is very new then it is unlikely to have small surface scratches inside it that provide a place for the bubbles to form. As the bubbles cannot form and release some of the heat that has built up, the liquid does not boil, and the liquid continues to heat up well past its boiling point. What then happens is that the liquid is bumped or jarred, which is just enough of a shock to cause the bubbles to rapidly form and expel the hot liquid. The rapid formation of bubbles is also why a carbonated beverage spews when opened after having been shaken. So please be very careful heating plain water in a microwave oven.

Enuf said!

Dear Dr. Ressel

I would just like to take a minute to tell you how meeting you has changed our lives. After a three-year roller coaster ride of falling through the cracks of our traditional health care system, I was reduced to a pill-popping patient plagued with side effects of the drug treatment I was under.

In November, my wife, children, and I attended a Natural Wellness Exhibit at the Botanical Gardens and while my wife and children toured the exhibits, I sat in on a lecture given by you. You talked about the spine and how the vertebras intertwine with the nerves and how it affects every part of our bodies. Our whole wellbeing is based on nerve energy. Then you began speaking of children's cases you could relate to. I have known other excellent chiropractors but you had a very different approach.

Shortly thereafter, my family and I got full assessments and began regular visits. My health has improved continually and my wife's migraines are an infrequent thing now. Your true joy and happiness are the children and your relationship with all the children seems to feed your passion for life in general. My children's general health is much better and they seem more resistant colds and flus and every day tribulations. My family is enjoying an overall sense of good health.

Patient First Chiropractic and Wellness Centre is not only a chiropractic clinic but a Center run by a man who is genuinely interested in the overall well being of his patients. The clinic is focused, and you encourage all your staff to attend seminars and lectures, and you make the information available to us. The overall atmosphere of your clinic encourages everyone to focus on overall well being based on chiropractic principles. We are all grateful.

My whole family graciously thanks you for your insight and dedication to your work. The articles and all the information you bring to us has been very helpful to the betterment of our overall health care. We have all been patiently looking forward to having your work bound for home reference. Your approach is very unique and we all benefit knowing you.

God Bless.

-The Boncori Family

6. Infertility

One of the most devastating problems facing many couples today is not being able to have a child, i.e. Infertility. I see this in many patients that I have had the good fortune to meet. The anguish is nothing short of heart- breaking, for many such couples have done everything – fertility clinics, fertility enhancing drugs, vitamin injections, counseling, etc. all to no avail.

In my own experience, I have found most cases of infertility to be fairly one-sided. In other words, I have found that it is usually women that seem to be at fault and unable to achieve pregnancy. Now, do not get me wrong, I am not blaming women for this difficulty in any way. This is not a sexist remark, but the problem, as I have observed, seems to be more allied with women than with men. Let me explain.

Women are much more familiar with reproductive function than most men. For you who are not all that aware of exactly how this all takes place, let's look at the following. When a woman ovulates, the egg travels down one Fallopian tube one month, and then down the other Fallopian tube the next month. In other words, it tends to alternate to give one or the other a "break." The egg starts at one end of the Fallopian tube and ends up at the uterus or womb at the other. The egg does not swim or have any flippers, arms, or legs, and so it is carried along by what we call passive transport. In other words, it is simply a bystander going for a ride; much like a ride in a convoluted water tube of a water park.

The reason this takes place is because of a very exact function of the different muscles that make up the walls of the Fallopian tubes. They literally "squeeze" the egg from one end of the tube to the other. The purpose of this function is to meet the sperm at the other end so that fertilization can take place. In other words, the egg starts at one end of the Fallopian tube and the muscles of the tube gently propel it from one end to the other. This process is called *peristalsis* and is very similar to swallowing while you eat – the muscles in your esophagus, the tube which you swallow food through, literally guide what you have just swallowed all the way down into your stomach. The same is true for the Fallopian tube.

Let's look at this in the light of a couple not being able to achieve pregnancy. In most couples who are labeled "INFERTILE" (and you know how much I detest labels), it seems that the egg is not able to make it through the Fallopian tube to meet the sperm. Unless that union is allowed to take place, there is no pregnancy, hence no baby – not a good thing.

We can look at this even closer. As I mentioned, the function of the muscles of the Fallopian tubes is to propel the egg from one end to the other, in order to meet the sperm. In cases of Infertility, however, this does not take place. Why would the muscles that are *designed* and *programmed* to perform that very special function every month, suddenly decide that they simply won't do it? Well, the answer is quite simple. It is not their decision. The muscles of your body do not decide what to do on their own.

They are literally ordered or not ordered to do their job. In cases of Infertility, I have found that the muscles are simply not able to take the egg from one end of the Fallopian tube to the other. In most cases, it is the fault of the nervous system, which controls that very function. The muscles of the Fallopian tubes either receive proper input from the nervous system to do their job, or they do not. In those cases I have found that the culprit is a vertebral subluxation, generally in the lower part of the spine, which interferes with the manner in which the Fallopian tubes would normally function.[34] Consider this similar to being on your cell phone – your reception and transmission suddenly being poor – you are not receiving your message. (I wrote a research paper on this which was published in December, 2004.)

By correcting the subluxation and allowing the nervous system to be then able to control the function of those Fallopian tubes normally, I have found that couples can achieve pregnancy. As "proof" that this theory actually works very well, we have a number of children

---

[34] Ressel, Ogi, Infertility: A Commentary, JVSR, December, 2004.

running around our Centre who are living proof and testimony of the amazing power of the body to function normally.

I simply must tell you of a story which you may find humorous – at my expense.

I was looking after a young 26 year old woman who came to see me with being unable to get pregnant. I placed her on a schedule of care designed to correct the Vertebral Subluxations which were at the root of her problem.

One day, she waltzed into our Centre with an amazing smile on her face. I want you to picture this for a moment – it is Friday morning, all the chairs in our reception area are full, the office is packed with people, and I am some 40 feet away from the front door. This patient stood in the doorway, joy on her face, arms outstretched, and yelled out: "You got me pregnant!"

There wasn't a sound in the office – no one moved. Needless to say, I had a lot of explaining to do!

I am including a letter from one of my patients that you will probably find quite interesting. It is just another example of Innate at work!

* * *

Dear Dr. Ressel:

We are sending you this letter to show our appreciation for all the help you have given us since we met you three years ago. Karen and I did not realize just what an impact "The Chiropractic Approach" would have on our lives.

After being married ten years, and trying to have a family for at least seven years, we had almost given up on the possibility. After four to five years of not taking birth control pills and not getting pregnant, Karen purchased a book on infertility. It had suggested charting Karen's basal body temperature each day. After eight months of continuous charting, the family doctor sent her to the gynecologist. He reviewed the charts, semen-analysis (lower count and motility, but that should not have been a problem) and decided to do a Laparoscopy (surgery to check the fallopian tubes). The surgery showed a couple of fibroids but they should not have been a problem.

The next step was to do Artificial Insemination in the gynecologist's office along with fertility drugs. No luck with the four attempts at Artificial Insemination and drugs. We were about to be referred to a Fertility Clinic when we bought our home in Burlington. At that time, family was not a priority so the Fertility Clinic was put on hold.

Just five months later we would meet you and you explained that Karen has a spinal curvature that could be causing her painful menstrual cycle and preventing pregnancy. Just six months after Karen started having adjustments, we got the news. On May 5, 1998, we were blessed with our first child, Cassie, weighing 7 lbs., 5 oz. Then on March 2, 2000, our son Timothy was born weighing 9 lbs., 3 oz.

We firmly believe these blessed events could not have been achieved without your help. Both children were born healthy and continue to enjoy good health due to regular adjustments and no vaccinations.

Our lives have been practically drug free in the past three years since you explained that our bodies can heal themselves. We can only hope that more people will follow the Chiropractic approach to better health. We will continue to be adjusted and help spread the word of a drug free lifestyle.

-Sandy & Karen Goldsmith

If you or someone you know is having difficulty achieving pregnancy, I strongly suggest they consult a chiropractor for an opinion first, before time is wasted on seeking some new wonder drug or therapy.

7. Baby Talk

So you just found out you're pregnant. Congratulations! That is wonderful! What is even more amazing is that your baby already has a spine, most of its body organs, arms and legs beginning to form, and its own nervous system. And it's only five weeks old! Miraculous! In order for your baby to develop normally, it has two basic needs; one is a normally operating nervous system, and the other is proper nutrition. Let's cover nutrition first.

Some people operate under the impression that as long as they are not hungry, they eat nutritiously. Not true! As a mom, you must be aware that *everything* you eat and drink affects your baby. Everything! Generally the baby will take from the mother whatever it needs in terms of nutrition. As a result, I have met many mothers in my practice who are literally undernourished. As a mom, you must remember that you are "eating for two. "Simply "filling up" is not the answer.

Your baby has very specific needs as it is growing and developing. Its rate of growth is *seven times faster* than its three-year-old brother. Much like feeding a baby elephant! It is, therefore, important that mom provides proper fuel for all that rapid growth. The following are *essential* for normal development of your baby:

1. **Iron:** Mom requires at least 800 mg daily. This is crucial for the development of red blood cells in your baby and is contained in most dark leafy veggies. You can also obtain a liquid iron supplement from your health food store. The nicest way of getting iron though is from a tablespoon of dark molasses in a glass of milk three times a day. What a way to treat your baby! Taking vitamin C will also help in the absorption of iron from your digestive tract.

2. **Folic Acid:** Very important in the normal development of the nervous system and cannot be omitted. After all, the nervous system is responsible for how your baby develops – so get with the program! You are lucky though. Folic Acid is contained in most foods that contain iron so it's a cinch to get. If you really want to get fancy, oysters are loaded with Folic Acid. They are also a known aphrodisiac and that may be why you are reading this chapter, but then that is another topic!

3. **Calcium:** Our friend! Mom and baby need at least 1200mg daily. The molasses treat is a good way to get some Calcium into your system and so is cheese, dairy foods, etc., or you may try raw almonds if you are not into dairy. It is important to know that Vitamin D helps in the absorption of Calcium from the digestive tract. In children this is easy – they absorb Vitamin D from the foods they eat. However, adults can't do this. In the adult, the absorption of Vitamin D is in the pitiful range but the adult skin manufactures Vitamin D when exposed to sunlight. So all those Caribbean vacations you have been dreaming about are actually nutritionally good for you! I found that the easiest way of getting Vitamin D is from a careful suntan, whether it is outside or in a reputable tanning salon. If you do decide to use the "electric beach," be careful of heat. Babies do not like getting too hot!

A word of caution for moms taking Vitamin B6 when pregnant: it tends to reduce the amount of breast milk available for feeding – not a good thing! And while I'm on the subject, babies do not like garlic, so avoid Caesar salads, etc., while breast-feeding. As well, chocolate gives babies diarrhea. This is a tough one as I have found that chocolate seems to be an indispensable staple for most moms.

I would like to address some of the taboos and misunderstandings often associated with moms being pregnant. One of the biggest is this whole issue of weight gain. Moms all over the world secretly look in the mirror and cringe at the sight of the loss of their waist, their "fat" stomach, enlarged breasts, swollen feet, and the fact that they often carry drips of their lunch on their T-shirt. Let me be emphatic here: You are not FAT, you are PREGNANT!! Huge difference! Swelling is actually a sign of a healthy pregnancy, not something that should be treated. Retention of fluids is healthy for mom and baby. It is also temporary. Just part of being pregnant!

A generation ago, weight gain was limited to eight to ten pounds. It was soon discovered that moms and babies were undernourished so the magic number became 24. This is no longer the case. Latest research indicates that weight gain of 35 lbs. or more on a high protein diet is healthy, as long as it is well balanced, does not contain chemicals or preservatives, and is limited in refined sugars.

The other issue revolves around salt. Moms are often told to re-strict their salt intake because of the secret fear of water retention, which then increases weight (here we go again). You should realize that sodium (a part of salt) is very important in the production of extra blood volume, which is essential for a growing baby, and a lack of it can be disastrous. I recommend that you use salt to "taste" and no more. This is an easy way to listen to what your body is telling you. If you suddenly have a craving for potato chips – go for it – your body is talking to you.

There are other no-no's you should be aware of when you're pregnant. One is alcohol. It causes problems with the development of your baby's nervous system. Caffeine is another and can be found in coffee, cola, black and green teas, and chocolate, and has been linked to birth defects. As well, try to limit your preservative intake including aspartame (refer to my chapter entitled, "Poisoning your Children"). Your baby will thank you later. Be very cautious using any type of drugs or medications. All have adverse effects on your baby. I should be emphatic here – *all drugs* cross the placental barrier and affect your baby. There is no such thing as a safe drug.

One of the most common nuisances of pregnancy is this "morning sickness" thing. Most of this is caused by a lack of blood sugar in the mother, i.e. hypoglycemia. After all, you have not eaten since 7–8:00 p.m. the night before, and your developing baby is literally feeding all night while you are asleep. Your blood sugar level is dangerously low by morning and you feel sick. I ask my patients to have an energy bar or a snack high in protein, fructose, and complex carbohydrates late in the evening, which will level out their blood sugar until breakfast – very simple, but very effective.

There are a number of things you can do to make your pregnancy the enjoyable experience it was meant to be. Commit to having a chiropractic check up to make sure your nervous system is functioning normally. This may assure you have a good pregnancy and much easier labour and delivery. Chiropractic for pregnancy has little to do with back pain, but is crucial for optimal health. I feel this is a must in having a healthy pregnancy.

The use of herbs such as red raspberry leaves makes for a good uterine tonic, and helps prevent miscarriage, anemia, and aids in fighting infection. Peppermint tea will help with digestion and nausea – so will ginger root. Other herbs such as Echinacea and chamomile are very relaxing and should be taken as a hot tea. Some people are concerned about Echinacea taken while you are pregnant. There are a number of conflicting opinions on this, but I've never encountered a mom having a problem with it – or any adverse effects on the baby. All these are available from your health food store.

Your family chiropractor will be invaluable in providing you with sound advice, which is not based on allopathic principles.

I just had to include this tid-bit:

"Mama got the rhythm, baby got the beat."
A new study says that's the reason women all over the world bounce, rock and jiggle their babies while they sing to them – it's helping to introduce a sense of rhythm. It may also be an early step in

the development of music appreciation, says the study by researchers at McMaster University, released today in the journal *Science*, an article in the Toronto Star reported.

The researchers wanted to test the idea that movement influences how the infant brain processes music – and it does.

So ... babies were born to boogie![35]

---

[35] Carey Elaine, Babies Truly Born to Boogie, Toronto Star, June 3, 2005.

8. Traumatic Birth Syndrome

This is a very disturbing topic and one that is unfamiliar to most parents. Traumatic Birth Syndrome (TBS), estimated to be the sixth leading cause of infant death, is mostly under reported and misdiagnosed. And of course your doctor will not have any clue, if you mention the subject.

Birth is a very normal biological process. It does not require "management" as a disease, yet most physicians and hospitals treat it in the manner of a sickness – much to the alarm of parents.

Both pregnancy and birth have special significance to a pediatric chiropractor – often a pregnant mom and child are exposed to harmful routine medical procedures that are not only poorly researched but whose effects are also not well documented. Most parents simply trust their doctor and that's it. This blind, simplistic view of birth can be life threatening to an infant.

My concern, when dealing with pregnancy, is the status of mom's spine and nervous system so that she can maintain a healthy pregnancy – it is important that all neural relays and connections are working optimally. This will ensure a mom to have a good, uneventful delivery resulting in a healthy baby. The reason is that vertebral subluxations often can affect a mother's spine causing malfunction, changing the physiology of pregnancy, and affecting the baby in-utero.

How you ask? An interference in the function of mom's nervous system will affect the manner in which the baby rotates and turns in the womb, for example. It will also affect baby's nutrition, development, and hence their growth. These factors can lead to what is called *In-Utero Constraint*. This is a situation where, in the last trimester of pregnancy, the baby is trapped in a precarious position in the Uterus, from which it is unable to free itself. This can lead to serious consequences during birth. For example; of the baby is trapped in what is called a "transverse lie" – a horizontal position across the uterus – it will most likely be born with a considerable Scoliosis – curvature of the spine. This may necessitate a long-term correction with your chiropractor. Or the baby is trapped with the his head in extension – resting on the back of his shoulders. This may cause problems with his spinal cord, etc. It is for this reason that I feel very strongly all pregnant moms should have a check up with a chiropractor to help them and their babies through their pregnancy, delivery, and birth.

I have mentioned previously alcohol consumption by mom and its effect on the development of the baby's nervous system. I did not mention smoking. Although a pregnant mom may decide not to smoke, she and her baby may be exposed to the toxic effects of second-hand smoke at work, home, etc. The fetus can receive second-hand smoke and evidence suggests low birth weight, as well as body malformations can be the result. As a mater of fact, many authorities feel that second-hand smoke is more dangerous.

As well, many women take over-the-counter medications during their pregnancy and do not question their safety. The feeling seems to be that if it is not prescribed then it is "safe." Let me be emphatic here. *All drugs affect your baby!* Most effects have not even been researched yet. The safety of prescribed medications on the fetus has not been researched but it is well documented that in the adult population, properly prescribed medications are the *third leading cause of preventable death!* Get real!

Why am I spending so much time on this subject? The answer is simple. Traumatic Birth Syndrome (TBS) accounts for 85–95 percent of health problems chiropractors see even in adults. Yes! Believe it or not, this is a huge problem. During the process of delivery, there is tremendous stress placed on the head and neck of the baby and often this stress causes vertebral subluxations of the very delicate spinal bones of the infant. This, in turn, affects the spinal cord and parts of the nervous system of the baby and can produce a myriad of health problems. These can appear seemingly unrelated to the process of delivery and can affect your child months or years later – even as an adult!

As I mentioned earlier in this chapter, Traumatic Birth Syndrome is a problem largely under-reported, and one that most people are unfamiliar with. Drs. G. Gutmann[36] and H. Biederman,[37] two German physicians, have done extensive studies on this phenomenon and found that in cases of subluxation generally of the neck area, the baby can literally stop breathing while asleep. This has been termed Sudden Infant Death Syndrome (SIDS).

A subluxation in the upper part of the neck area, usually from the process of delivery, affects the spinal cord.[38] In that particular area of the spinal cord, called the brain stem, are located the centers for breathing. In other words, these are the areas that control whether a person breathes or not. A subluxation in that area can then affect these breathing centers causing a baby to literally stop breathing. Not a good thing!

Dr. Gutmann also found that 80 percent of all children tend to have a subluxation in the upper part of the neck, which may make them susceptible to a number of diffuse symptoms which have baffled physicians for years. He also found that this type of subluxation could also cause lower resistance to infection, frequent colds, ear problems, hyperactivity, Asthma, bed-wetting, as well as what he termed, "central motor impairment." His recommendation to parents is that "a spinal check up after birth should be obligatory." This is so important that certain hospitals in Australia are now having chiropractors check infants immediately after delivery to ensure a healthy spine and nervous system free from subluxations. I think this is a wonderful idea.

Do you think this would ever become commonplace in North America? I can almost hear you say: Why is this so important?

I mentioned earlier that your child's spine is her/his lifeline. Running through it is the spinal cord containing billions of nerves that send vital messages and information from the brain to every part of the body and back again. Yes, we all have our own internal Internet! As long as none of these messages are interrupted, your child should have optimal

---

[36] Gutman, G., *Blocked Atlantal Nerve Syndromes in Babies and Infants*, Manuelle Medizin, 1987, 25, 5-10.

[37] Biederman, H., "Kinematic Imbalances Due to Suboccipital Strain in Newborns,"*Journal Manual Medicine*, 1992; 6:151-156.

[38] Towbin, A., "Latent Spinal Cord and Brain Stem Injury in Newborn Infants," *Medical Child Neurology*, 1969, 11, 54-68.

function and the best of health! If, however, there is an interference with this "information highway," such as a vertebral subluxation, the messages sent by the brain will not reach the part of the body they are intended to reach. As a result, the body begins to work improperly. This is "malfunction." It can be a serious threat to health. This interference will also affect your baby's immune system, lower body resistance and leave your child prey to various "bugs" and infections. Often parents would ask me: "Why is it that my child always seems to be sick?" How many of you have a child who seems to get "everything" while your other children seems to be really healthy? ... And you have been told that this child has a "weak" constitution. What does that mean – exactly?

In cases such as these, the problem is that in all likelihood, the child has had a difficult birth and is presently suffering from Vertebral Subluxations – his body is not functioning as it should!

I feel that as a parent you should be aware of information well accepted, recognized, and deeply rooted medical procedures and rituals, that may contribute to Traumatic Birth Syndrome, thereby affecting the health of your baby – even for life:

1. ***Ultrasound.*** The first of these is *"Ultrasound."* This procedure, many think, seems "safe" and innocuous. Current research, however, tells us that this is not so. First of all, ultrasound tends to cause an error in the way cells function. Diagnostic ultrasound causes genetic damage and alterations in cellular growth and function. It also plays havoc with the cell genetic code. This means that it is possible to create errors in the very Code that make your baby a Human Being. Not only that, but Ultrasound has also been associated with dyslexia and delayed speech as well as demyelination (Myelin is the covering which protects nerves and prevents 'short-circuits') of the brain – not a good thing! This last effect was the result of a study done using rats. I'll let you draw your own conclusions though.

This next interesting tid-bit is from *The Sunday Telegraph*, Dec. 10, 2001:[39]

LONDON - Swedish scientists have uncovered evidence suggesting that ultrasound scans on pregnant women can cause brain damage in their unborn babies. In the most comprehensive study yet on the effects of the scanning, a team of doctors found that men born to mothers who underwent scanning were more likely to show signs of subtle brain damage.

During the 1990s, a number of studies hinted that ultrasound scanning affected unborn babies. Research has suggested that subtle brain damage can cause people who ought genetically to be right-handed to become left-handed. In addition, these people face a higher risk of conditions ranging from learning difficulties to epilepsy. The findings would mean that ultrasound scans are causing slight brain damage in thousands of babies each year.

Ultrasound scans, which were introduced in the 1960s, have long been regarded as a safe means of checking on the health of unborn children. The scanners use high-frequency sound waves to give X-ray-like images of the inside of the womb. According to the Swedish researchers, the human brain undergoes critical development until relatively late in pregnancy, making it vulnerable to damage. In addition, the male brain is especially at risk, as it continues to develop later than the female brain.

Beverley Beech, the chairwoman of Britain's Association for Improvements in Maternity Services, criticized doctors for insisting for years that ultrasound was totally safe. "I am not sure at all that the benefits of ultrasound scans outweigh the downsides," Ms. Beech said.

---

[39] Matthews, Robert, "Ultrasound Linked to Brain Damage," The Sunday Telegraph, Dec 10, 2001.

"We should be advising women to think very, very carefully before they have scans at all."

Of greatest concern, however, is the fact that ultrasound affects the immature eggs of a female baby thus affecting her own children. Because this technology is relatively new, this last effect has not been investigated thoroughly, but parents everywhere should beware!

2. ***Electronic Fetal Monitoring (EFM).*** This used by most hospitals although there has been little testing done to determine its efficacy. Latest research does indicate that it increases parent panic and has increased C-sections by 400 percent. There is nothing more chilling for parents to hear during delivery than the words, "the baby's heart rate is dropping." This is the point where all logic leaves and panic takes over. Many moms do not realize that it is quite normal for the heart rate of the baby to drop slightly during each contraction. **THIS IS NORMAL!!!** However panic will ensure total compliance by parents to any and all hospital procedures and rituals. Wonderful for the hospital's bottom line!

3. ***Epidurals.*** This has been shown to increase labour time and cause fever in the mother, which is then treated with antibiotics for both mom and baby. Brilliant! As well, it does not allow the mother to "feel" her labour, which then necessitates the use of forceps, vacuum extraction, and even C-section to deliver the baby.

4. ***Forceps and Vacuum extraction.*** These procedures use up to 140 lbs. of force to literally pull the baby "out." These are the main two that cause most of the health problems seen in children and even adults. The forces

applied to the head and neck of the baby often cause nerve and spinal cord injuries as well as vertebral subluxations. These subluxations affect the baby's nervous system and are a great threat to health not only immediately, but can affect the health of that child even into adulthood.

As well, forceps-assisted childbirth significantly boosts a woman's risk of fecal incontinence. Approximately 10 percent of moms report experiencing fecal incontinence during the year following childbirth. Those whose deliveries involved forceps and who experienced tears in the anal sphincter were at double the risk of fecal incontinence during the three months following delivery, compared with mothers whose deliveries did not involve forceps. So ... the moral of this story is to give this much thought before allowing forceps top be used.

5. ***Caesarean sections.*** These have been increasingly popular with the advent of EFM, Amniocentesis, and Chorionic Villi sampling. It seems to be presented as a very simple procedure, yet many parents do not realize that it *IS* surgery. As soon as the abdomen is cut, the uterus tends to contract to protect the baby. This often necessitates the use of steel retractors to open the uterus, then forceps and vacuum extraction to deliver the baby. Of course, the mother is anesthetized so she can't feel pain. Many forget that the anesthetic that mom is given, also crosses the placenta and affects the baby. Definitely not the birth of choice! This seems to be used increasingly by most hospitals as the preferred method of delivery, for it provides a hospital with a definite date and time of delivery – the baby is born at a prearranged time.

No one is inconvenienced and no golf games are thus interrupted. What great convenience!

Another tid-bit that I'll share with you is that natural childbirth may prevent a baby from developing Asthma later in life – a recent study followed 1,953 Finnish subjects from their birth in 1966 to their third decade in life in 1997. The 5.3 percent of subjects who were delivered via Cesarean section were three times more likely to have developed asthma by age 31, compared with subjects delivered vaginally.

And while I'm on the subject, let's talk about Pitocin, the synthetic hormone used in order to stimulate delivery. Are there problems with the use of Pitocin? Yes!

Oxytocin, your body's natural hormone, is secreted in bursts. However, when you are given pitocin you are placed on a regulated intravenous pump, to regulate the amount of pitocin to a steady flow. Therefore, pitocin induced contractions are entirely different from your body's natural contractions, in both strength and effect.

With pitocin, the induced force of the contraction may decrease uterine blood flow (this is also done during a natural contraction, but not for as long of a period and not as close together) therefore, reducing the oxygen to the baby. You will also receive continuous electronic fetal monitoring with pitocin. This is because fetal distress is more common with pitocin use and needs to be detected if it occurs. I'll bet this makes you feel better already! Pitocin can be the first domino in the domino effect. The IV, the infusion pump, and the continuous monitoring will confine most moms to bed, decreasing her ability to deal with her contractions naturally. With the more painful contractions, a mother is more likely to need pain medication, such as an epidural anaesthesia – I have already discussed this above

Pitocin can present other hazards. For the mother these include: turbulent labor and contractions – which may cause early separation of the placenta (placenta previa), rupture of the uterus, lacerations of the cervix or post birth hemorrhage. Fetal hazards include: fetal asphyxia and neonatal hypoxia from too frequent and prolonged uterine contractions, physical injury and premature delivery if the due date is not accurate.

You may not be aware of this but a class action lawsuit has been filed in Tennessee against the manufacturer of Pitocin that has been used on millions of pregnant women to stimulate contractions during childbirth.[40]

The drug is Pitocin, and the lawsuit alleges that it is "dangerously defective" and may be linked to the deaths of several mothers during childbirth and health problems with some babies. One doctor said he was "shocked" at the news of the lawsuit. "I'm sure someone has a legitimate concern, but this is really surprising to me, "Dr. Peter Mark said, "All the hospitals, obstetricians and gynecologists use it almost every day. I wouldn't know how to practice without it, it's useful." Marks did say that the drug can sometimes be overused. The lawsuit alleges that the drug itself isn't causing the problems; rather it is a preservative in the mixture called cholobutanol that lawyers are alleging causes the dangerous side effects. In addition to possibly causing deaths of mothers during childbirth, some suggest its use may be linked to autism in some babies and low oxygen levels in others. Manufacturers of the drug say there are some health risks for some women given the drug, but defends both as well as its labelling.

I'll bet you are feeling better already.

The greatest difficulty Doctors of Chiropractic have with all these procedures is that they lead to the increased possibility of vertebral subluxations in the baby's spine—not a good thing! By now, you have probably guessed that I feel it is imperative to have babies checked for subluxations as soon as possible after birth.

You are probably thinking; "So what is my alternative?" Well, I have always been a proponent of Home Birth. Many moms may feel a bit uneasy about having their baby at home – relax you are not alone – nor will you be alone during your delivery. Amazingly knowledgeable and competent midwives will be assisting you. This headline appeared on

---

[40] Lemay Gloria; Childbirth Drug Pitocin is Lawsuit Target, www.obgyn.net, Feb 23, 2001, 20:29:08 2001.

Feb. 6, 2002 on online Web MD: *"Home Births Safe for Most."* It reported on the February 5, 2002 study published in the Canadian Medical Association Journal. In this study researchers compared the outcomes of 862 planned home births attended by midwives with those of planned hospital births attended by either midwives (571) or physicians (743) during the years 1998 and 1999.[41]

The results of the study showed that women who gave birth at home attended by a midwife had fewer procedures during labor compared with women who gave birth in a hospital attended by a physician. The study also suggests that home births have a lower incidence of infection and use of drugs for pain. Additionally, women in the home birth group were less likely to have epidural analgesia, have their labor induced, or have an episiotomy.

And as far as the overall safety of home births, the researchers concluded that the number of deaths was similar to that found in other studies and the difference in death rate between the two groups was too small to be statistically important. The conclusions of the researchers as published in the journal were as follows: *"Interpretation: There was no increased maternal or neonatal risk associated with planned home birth under the care of a regulated midwife. The rates of some adverse outcomes were too low for us to draw statistical comparisons, and ongoing evaluation of home birth is warranted. There was no increased maternal or neonatal risk associated with planned home birth under the care of a regulated midwife,"* the authors wrote.

In a commentary article in the same issue, Régis Blais, MD, from the Université de Montréal, agrees that this *"study provides valuable information about the safety of home birth that should help expectant parents make their choice of place of birth and caregiver."*

So there you have it!

* * *

---

[41] "Home Births Safe for Most," *Web MD*, February 6, 2002.

Dear Dr. Ressel,

Four years ago, my husband and I were blessed with the safe arrival of our son, Riley. I mention safe, because Riley came very close to not surviving. After a few days in intensive care, our son fought for his life with everything that he had.

He has grown to become a very intelligent, warm and active little boy. Riley was born with Down Syndrome. If you look in any medical journal for a perspective on this syndrome, you will find that the information is very limited, and the picture painted is not a pretty one. We were immediately in contact with a whole host of professionals, doctors/ specialists and support groups. Although most were trying to be supportive, they seemed to have this complicated attitude, "Accept your son for whatever he can or can't do, make the best of it." Whenever we would question something medically, we were often met with a puzzled look, "Well it's because he has Down Syndrome," but no one could explain why this was occurring. Well I have come to understand this is simply because they don't know. What was very obvious to me was that these professionals seemed to be only dealing with the symptoms of the problem. They were not looking beyond the label, as to why this was occurring. And so began our quest to unravel the mystery behind the syndrome. It wasn't long before we found many people who were on similar journeys. Silly me, I thought I could take this information back to the same professionals to share my new findings. Need I say more? I got several blank stares, was told I was in denial, and some doctors even tried the intimidation approach. Needless to say, I did not have a lot of trust or respect for the resources available to me.

A dear friend, who, knowing my philosophy and experiences introduced me to Dr. Ogi Ressel. I had a limited and somewhat skeptical view of chiropractic care, but decided I would at least hear what this doctor had to say. I was not willing to subject my son to yet another professional and so I decided I would make the appointment for myself and just bring my son along.

My first visit to the clinic was like nothing I had experienced before. I was greeted by the staff who treated me as though I was a long, lost relative. They put a movie on for my son to occupy him and even offered to watch over him while I had my visit. This was a far cry from the usual doctor's office where you have a forty-five minute wait. I happened to be in the last stages of my next pregnancy at that point, and through a brief examination, Dr. Ressel was able to explain to me more about my pregnancy than any doctor I have ever been involved with previously.

It turned out that he was dead on about when I would give birth, even though I thought he was way off. He helped me to change my mind-set about the entire birthing process, which I will be eternally grateful for. He talked to me as an equal, not only asked my opinion, but also actually cared about what I had to say; he even offered me his home phone number. Unheard of! I walked out of that appointment with all kinds of material and the feeling that I only wished I had learned about this earlier, particularly for my pregnancy. But the thing that impressed me most was his attitude towards Riley. His emphasis was on Riley as a four-year-old and the problems he was experiencing. It wasn't until the latter part of the conversation that he mentioned the fact that Riley had Down Syndrome. I was so taken aback by this that I didn't know what to think. I was almost suspicious, but I knew that underlying all of this, I have made an important discovery.

Riley is a very intuitive person. He can detect if people are genuine or not, and I have come to rely on and respect his judgement of people. He usually resists going to doctor's and being poked and prodded, but he took to Dr. Ressel, or as he calls him "Ogi," right away.

Shortly after my daughter was born, she was experiencing a mild case of colic, enough to keep us sleep deprived. The doctors said there was nothing we could do. It was my midwife who mentioned the option of chiropractic care. I decided to bring her to see "Ogi" as well. Within a week and a half the colic was gone, most importantly, my daughter seemed to be so much more content and alert. Not only did he help my daughter, but this allowed me the opportunity to see him in action and acquire a greater appreciation for the passion that this man brings to his work. The way he handled my daughter was as if she were his own.

Even with all of those results it was still hard for me to allow Dr. Ressel to care for Riley. Subconsciously, I think I was trying to find reasons not to bring my son, but Dr. Ressel just kept giving me that gentle nudge. It took several weeks of my questioning and at times interrogation, but he was always willing to take the time to listen, often calling me from his home in the evening after clinic hours. It took time but we had now built a solid trusting partnership, and I knew that there was a great deal of knowledge and integrity behind Dr. Ressel's work. Once we had the special x-rays done that Dr. Ressel needed, it was confirmed that Riley had acquired quite a number of subluxations in the top part of his spine, which were having a dramatic impact on the functioning of his central nervous system. This was something both Dr. Ressel and I have suspected. It has only been a short time since Riley has started to see Dr. Ressel, and I am not expecting overnight result. But for the first time in a long time, I feel like I am doing everything in my power to ensure my children are the healthiest they can be. I can't help but wonder how other children might benefit from this type of care.

In the U.S. last year one million more children were prescribed Ritalin. In the last ten years there has been 40 percent increase in the labelling of children. Astonishing! Are we dealing with symptoms or the underlying cause? I think I know the answer to that one.

I commend Dr. Ressel for the work he is doing, and only hope that others will be open enough to hear his message.

-Leanne Kirk

9. Infantile Colic

Of all the health challenges that seem to plague infants, this is probably the one that causes most upset with parents. Imagine for a moment feeding your child, when all of a sudden he/she begins screaming at the top of their lungs, arms curling in, legs drawing up, with what seems to be agonizing pain. All the common remedies associated with "over-the-fence" and grandmotherly advice seem to be of no avail. Colic and ear infections are the two that tug at mothers and fathers' heartstrings more than any other condition that I saw at our Center.

Most textbooks describing Colic mention that it usually happens in the evening hours. I have not found that to be the case. I found that it tends to occur at any time of the day and seems to have no rhyme or reason. Colic, it seems, tends to start sometime in infancy, around the first two weeks of life, and can persist for a number of months.

For those who are not familiar with Infantile Colic, and have never had the pleasure of dealing with a child who is so afflicted, you have no idea how devastating it can be on parents' nerves. Why? It's characterized by constant crying, screaming, whining, pains in the stomach area, and acute irritability. (This is not *cute* irritability; this is *acute* irritability – big difference between the two.) The spells of crying can last for hours, and parents' nerves are shot at the end of such spells. This type of crying leads to aerophagia, which means the swallowing of air. This then causes distention or enlargement of the bowels, which then creates more pain, which creates more crying, which creates more air being swallowed, which then becomes a cycle. Colic is also characterized by passing an exorbitant amount of gas and abdominal distention, which simply means the stomach area is enlarged and bloated (this gas thing can be embarrassing when in public). As well, the infant does not appear to be ill, is gaining weight, and has a good appetite. If either of those is absent, then the incessant crying can be caused by a problem different from Colic.

I would suggest you consult your family chiropractor to provide you with advice.

There have been many theories people have used in the past to attempt to explain what Colic really is and why it occurs. Some authorities have blamed lactose intolerance; some felt it is caused by stress of the parents, stress of the baby, abnormal gall bladder function, higher levels of intestinal hormones, allergic reactions, digestive hormone instability, etc. None of these seem to be the problem. A just-published study confirms what many parents and chiropractors have long suspected: Colic is associated with allergy. Researchers in Finland tracked 116 infants for one week, at seven weeks of age, and for one week at 12 weeks of age. The study revealed that 38 percent of children who showed signs of allergies at 2 years of age were significantly more fussy during their seventh week and were more likely to have a colic-type cry during their twelfth week, compared with allergy-free babies. Much more study needs to be done on this association

One of the biggest concerns of a child having Colic is that there is a potential for possible child abuse. To be very frank, try to imagine a child screaming for hours, non-stop. I find that this will sometimes get on parents' nerves and on occasion we see a condition which is called "the shaken baby syndrome." This is a condition whereby the baby is literally shaken by the parents to somehow stop him/her from crying.

This only takes place when mom and dad are at their wit's end. But there is no excuse for this behavior. Shaking an infant can cause irreparable damage to a baby and even death. I am not suggesting that this is a huge problem, but there is potential for abuse of an infant who happens to be colicky. If you do ever feel that you as a parent are close to "losing it," remember that there is a reason this is taking place.

In my experience with dealing with thousands of children and babies, I found that often a vertebral subluxation in the spine affecting the way the nervous system controls bowel functions, is usually the cause of Colic. Any chiropractor involved in seeing children will attest to this fact. You must understand that the digestive system is essentially a long tube (refer to my chapter on Digestive Difficulties) and is made of muscle walls, which are under the direct control of the nervous system. I find that in the case of Colic, a vertebral subluxation will reduce the amount of information flowing from the brain to the large intestine, thereby reducing the normal function and motility of the large intestine. This causes food to "stick around" in the large intestine longer than it should and it tends to produce gas. This gas causes distention of the intestinal wall, causing pain and crying. The cry of the baby is really for help.

Children who are affected by Colic generally show a wonderful response in the hands of a chiropractor. Most often I find results within the first week of care, but the care must be directed at the correction of the subluxation which is at the root of the problem, not simply giving the child mere relief. If mere relief is given only, there is a very high possibility of the subluxation becoming chronic and then causing arthritic degeneration (refer to the chapter on Arthritis), later on in life – not a desirable situation. For those of you who have children affected by colic, I suggest you see a chiropractor without further delay. I am including a short letter from two young parents whose child was very badly affected with colic, to give you a sense of reality.

* * *

Dear Dr. Ressel,

Both my husband and I feel the need to express our gratitude toward your treatment of our son Lincoln. When we first brought him to you, he was only six weeks old and we had struggled for most of those weeks with his excessive gassiness, or what we though, might be colic. When everyone we spoke to told us this was normal and he would grow out of it. As a recent mother, I struggled with my feelings over this. As a new parent, it is a very scary feeling when you are helpless; not know-ing what is wrong with your child and no one can offer a suitable explanation. Although I knew there were many others in the same situation, I refused to believe that this was normal and acceptable. As his condition worsened, I stopped questioning my initial instincts and after a series of coincidences involving information on chiropractic, we decided to seek this alternative route of health care. Because we knew very little about chiropractic care, we did some research and the one aspect both my husband and I agreed upon, was that we wanted a specialist. That led us directly to you and here we are.

The first time we brought Lincoln to see you, we were told to open our mind and leave behind everything we perceived to be true   regarding standard health care. What we did not realize then, but do now, is how that was going to open up doors for us that we would have laughed at only weeks earlier. We are very skeptical at the best of times. Needless to say, after only a couple of weeks, our beautiful baby boy was actually acting like a child—happy and laughing. We have forgotten the long episodes of tears and screaming after his feedings. His gas is now gone, and he acts like a healthy infant, and very manageable. For this we would like to thank you.

I think what we appreciated most, was that not only did you treat our son with the care you would your own child, but that you took the time to fully explain in detail, all the possible causes and treatments of Lincoln's condition. I feel that it is very important for us to fully understand what was happening to our son. I now feel comfortable discussing the details of our story with other parents so that they too can realize that you do not need to just accept the fact that colic is normal and will run its course, which may be months. Because of all you have done, again thank you for enabling us to enjoy raising our new son, and we look forward to seeing you for our families' continued care over the years.

-Lori and Rohan Laylor

10. Dirt

You must be wondering about the title of this chapter and what could I possibly be thinking. Why such a crazy title? After all, you hate dirt! So do your family, friends and the vast majority of North Americans. We are obsessed with dirt and the unclean.

How many of you take off your shoes when entering the house, or look at a glass before drinking from it. Do you wash your hands compulsively, or wear a hospital gown while holding your newborn baby – it has more bacteria on it than your infant!

Why do we do this? Well, it is simple. We have been taught that germs are bad; that one can get germs from anything and everything; that germs should be eradicated, wiped out, killed, and that no mercy should be shown. We then pass this sterile obsession onto our children and the myth of clean is propagated.

This mentality is causing our own demise. More authorities are convinced that everyday dust and dirt are actually good for you. Our health is based on a properly functioning nervous system, immune system and the endocrine system. The new science connecting these components is called neuropsychoimmunology. Many feel that the immune system, the endocrine system, and the nervous system are one and the same. This new science investigates the relationships between these systems, and how they integrate and interact with each other for the health and well being of the individual.

Bart Classen, M.D. a vaccine researcher and President of Classen Immunotherapies in Maryland, a laboratory which sets out school vaccination schedules in the U.S., says that children's immune systems today are in serious trouble. He thinks that because of our search for cleanliness and sterility, our immune system is no longer being exercised as in the past. He also feels that our vaccination program is one of the leading causes of Asthma – more on that in a later chapter.[42] These thoughts are echoed by Dr. Stephen Marini, D.C.,

---

[42] Classen Bart, www.vaccines.net.

Ph.D., a chiropractor, immunologist, my friend, as well as Philip Incao, M.D., me, and countless others.

I can already hear one of you thinking; "You mean to tell me that the five second rule is actually true? When my son drops his toast on the floor, is it OK for him to still eat it?" My answer would simply be; "Most likely."

You may be surprised to learn that researchers in England are actually adding bacteria found in common everyday dirt to the diet of babies. The thinking is that it will stimulate their immune system for increased vigilance.

Chocolate or vanilla, anyone?

More and more scientists are realizing that most childhood diseases are quite innocuous, and are there in order to exercise a young and immature immune system. You probably think that a child having measles or chicken pox is a terrible thing – not so. These diseases actually teach the immune system how to deal with the myriad of viruses and bacteria. In fact, Dr. Howard Weiner, a prominent Harvard immunologist, thinks that our vaccination program actually skews the activity of the immune system; making our children more susceptible to more serious complications later in life. In these situations, an immature immune system will not be able to deal as effectively with a bacterial or viral invasion because it has never had to try. (I will discuss the issue of vaccination in considerable detail in another chapter.)

I used to tell my patients that even the common flu and cold has a place. They teach the immune system how to fight for survival. Just because you feel sick when you have the flu does not mean that you really are, it simply means that your body is doing exactly what it was programmed and designed to do. This is not sickness. This is an expression of health – your body is following its program. I am not saying that you have to like it though, but ultimately it is for your own benefit. To interfere with this function is not in your best interest. Dr. Phillip Incao, M.D., a Colorado phycian, agrees with this perception.

He feels that when you are really feeling "sick," you body is actually "cleaning house."[43]

Looking at this issue from a reality perspective though, there are a number of supplements I can recommend that will help your child's body increase the function of the immune system:

1. Vitamin B complex and magnesium
2. Antioxidants, such as Rhododendron caucasicum
3. Vitamin A
4. Zinc and Copper
5. Bovine colostrum and/or Echinacea
6. Garlic
7. Amino Acids (L-Arginine, L-Cystine, L-Lysine)

The other important point I would like to make is that the immune system is directly controlled by the nervous system. Therefore, it is absolutely imperative that you make sure your child is examined by a chiropractor, so that there are no vertebral subluxations affecting the way the nervous system transmits information. This will ensure normal and optimal nervous system and immune system function.

The point I am making is that our attitude toward dirt needs to change. So don't be so fastidious. Let some dirt into your life. Your children will be much happier and much healthier for it!

---

[43] Incao Phillip, "Not a Battle, But a Housecleaning," *Pathways*, ICPA, Issue 6, pg. 2.

11. Fever Frenzy

Your child is hot, flushed, glassy-eyed and obviously not well. As a mom (I am directing this specifically towards moms, because as I mentioned earlier, many dads defer to their wives as being responsible for the family's health care), your diagnosis is **FEVER**. You are very worried and concerned and can feel a little bit of panic setting in as well. After all, you have been carefully trained to think that fever is actually something that should be treated. You are probably thinking: "No, I haven't!" Think again. If you tune to any TV station at any time, or look at any popular magazine – even National Geographic – yes, they just succumbed to the almighty pharmaceutical dollar – you will most likely see a dozen or so commercials for anti-pyretic (anti-fever) medication. Aspirin – popular a few years ago and beginning to make a comeback, Tylenol, Children's Tylenol (what is that about?), as well as a host of others – all teaching you that fever is a bad thing – that if you want to be a good mom, you need to give these drugs to your family to combat this scourge of fever! What nonsense!

So, let's look at this fever thing for just a moment. We have been taught that normal body temperature hovers around 98.6 degrees Fahrenheit (37 degrees C). Right? Wrong! 98.6° F only represents an *average*. Your child's body temperature can hover anywhere between 97° F and 100°F and be considered "normal." Think of it. That's a lot of heat!

Let's take our bizarre thinking a step further. At what point does 98.6 degrees F become fever? Is it 99.0 degrees? Or 99.5? How about 99.8? When does it officially become fever? You see, there is no medical standard for this figure. So,- if 98.6 degrees doesn't worry a parent, why would 100°? There is not much difference between these two figures – only 1.4 degrees! If that is the case then, why is there such a panic throughout North America regarding a child who has a fever? I will get to the answer in a few moments.

We must realize that fever is just **HEAT**. Normal body temperature is the result of your child's body working as it was meant to, under the perfect control of the computer which runs each particular program – the nervous system; the heart pumping blood, normal respiration, normal breathing, normal digestive cycles, movement of different body muscles, etc. All these activities produce WORK and work produces HEAT. Although this is fairly simplified, in reality that is exactly what takes place. If that is the case, what is fever then?

To help your child recover when he or she is fighting a flu bug for example, the nervous systems demands an increase in heat production in order to literally "burn" invading germs (bacteria, virus), which can only survive at a "normal" body temperature. Any increase in heat, therefore, kills such invading organisms. This is a good thing.

As a result of orders from the nervous system, many body activities speed up. Respiration increases, the heart rate speeds up in order to pump blood faster, breathing increases, the skin is moist and clammy and the child begins to shiver, etc. Now, just as an aside, most people do not understand what shivering really is. Let me explain. Shivering is very rapid contraction of most of the body muscles in order to produce more work. And, more work produces ... you guessed it, more heat. When a child is shivering, it is not necessarily because he/she is cold. It is because the nervous system makes demands that the muscles contract, thereby increasing the work produced by the body. All of these, as well as many other bodily functions, are speeded up. This extra work produces *extra* heat. We call fever – simple!

If you look at all this extra activity, it has a purpose – to eliminate the invading germ and to restore normal health and order. Let me shatter another marketing myth. As soon as a child has a fever, we are automatically programmed to think that the child is SICK! When we acknowledge that our child is sick, we are then open to all sorts of drug remedies – wonderful for the drug company bottom line. Listen up ... When your child has a fever it does not necessarily mean that your child is "sick." After all, the body is doing what it has been programmed and designed to do. This is not "sick." This is an expression of health. How is that for a different perspective?

Let me give you an example of how miraculously your body functions. For instance, when a child has a respiratory infection, the flu or a cold, the breathing rate increases. The result of this is to provide extra oxygen for the body. With every extra breath your child takes in and exhales, the lungs actually get rid of the "bug," through the process of letting air out. Along with the stale air that comes out of your child's lungs, are millions of bacteria, viruses and other invading organisms.

Your child also has a loss of appetite, which is perfectly normal. The nervous system, in order to conserve energy and deal with the infection in a more efficient manner, shuts down the digestive process. Most of the body energy is then diverted to defense rather than assimilation of food. A cough is seen as another way of getting rid of the bacteria and viruses that have invaded his body. The skin is cold and clammy as a result of the increased sweating and perspiration – again designed to rid the body of the invading organism. Vomiting, diarrhea and nose drip are seen as the quickest way of getting rid of the virus and bacteria.

At the same time, the body temperature increases to what is generally considered above normal. At this stage, there may possibly be damage to the cornea of the eye, which is very heat sensitive. The body's protective measures call for a continuous washing of the eyes with tears, in order to cool down the cornea so there is no damage. Therefore, if you look at your child when he is considered "sick," the eyes will look very glassy.

As you can see from this explanation, this is really not "sickness." This is an expression of health. This is an expression of the innate wisdom of your child's body in knowing exactly what needs to be done at the right time and in the right amount.

Now, I never said you have to like it, but it is quite normal. This is also the point where most parents feel they have to "do something." Why? Because we have been taught that when a child is sick, we must intervene. Think about this for moment though. The most important thing here is to understand why this is happening, provide supportive care and *allow* your child's body to do what it needs to do all by itself *with no interference*. That can be tough! But think! The innate intelligence and wisdom that made your child from two cells to over 40 quadrillion in a matter of 280 days, knows exactly what that child needs, every time – as long as it is not interfered with. I don't think it is possible for that intelligence to suddenly abandon your child when he/she has the flu.

I want to interject for a moment – let's talk about the efficacy of OTM (over-the counter medication) before continuing on with our discussion on fever – seems like a perfect time to talk about this issue:

Researchers who studied a variety of over-the-counter cough medicines found no evidence that they provide any significant relief. The study, conduced by researchers at the University of Bristol in England, appeared in the British Medical Journal. Reviewed were 15 drug trials involving more that 2,000 patients that compared oral over-the-counter cough medicines with placebo in adults with acute cough. In nine trials, the drugs fared no better than placebo. The positive results in the other six studies were of *questionable* clinical relevance, said authors. Based on their study, the researchers concluded, "Over the counter cough medicines for acute cough cannot be recommended because there is no good evidence for effectiveness. Even when trials had significant results, the effect sizes were small and of doubtful clinical relevance." Cough medicines are widely available to the public without a medical prescription in most countries, and retail sales rose by $135 million between 1998 and 1999 in the United Kingdom alone.[44]

Back to our discussion of Fever – and it brings me to another point. The height (temperature) of a fever has really no bearing on the seriousness of the condition. There is no clinical evidence that suggests that a high fever causes convulsions or brain damage. Think about this for a moment. Why would the nervous system increase temperature to injure itself? It simply makes no sense. We have been carefully taught, however, to believe this is fact – old wives tales or an ingenious marketing plan? You decide.

Here is another ploy – why do you have to take your child's temperature when he/she is feverish? Good question – you don't.

---

[44] Schroeder Kurt, Fahey Tom, "Systematic review of randomised controlled trials of over the counter cough medicines for acute cough in adults," *British Medical Journal*, Feb. 9, 2002.

The degree of fever is not important. Increasing numbers of chiropractic doctors as well as physicians feel that a child's temperature should not be taken, and that taking a temperature is an unnecessary ritual. I could not agree more.

You are probably wondering that if this is the case, then how did this fever phobia begin? Well, it was borne out of marketing efforts by the pharmaceutical industry whose aim was to teach the public that fever should be feared and treated so that sales of antifever medications would soar. This marketing plan was very effective and is still prevalent today.

So, when is it necessary to treat fever? It isn't. It is neither necessary nor wise to lower body temperature. FEVER IS NOT THE PROBLEM: it is simply the result of the body attempting to recover. Any medications taken to lower the temperature of the body will work only temporarily. Once the body excretes them, the temperature will once again increase. The reason for this is that those drugs have no real effect on the problem and therefore giving them to your children changes nothing. I would suggest that you have your child checked by a chiropractor; the goal here would be to provide your child with the optimum function of the nervous system so that it could successfully deal with the "illness."

This may surprise you: I have just recently learned that back in the 1940s in Davenport, Iowa, many chiropractors of the time were referred to as "flu doctors" and apparently, many patients would see a chiropractor in those days when they had the flu. They found that the length of time of their illness, its severity and frequency was shortened sometimes up to 80 percent.

If you must absolutely do "something" while your child is recovering, there are a number of natural health products found in health food stores that may help your child cope with this period of time when the body is "doing its thing." There are, however, certain situations that warrant careful observation. If your child is under the age of one, and has a fever with the presence of any of the following signs, you should seek the advice of a health care professional: he/she is in severe pain and cannot be comforted, is anxious and or lethargic, whining continuously, cannot retain fluids and/or has diarrhea, has difficulty urinating, breathing, or swallowing, has an unexplained rash and has a rapid pulse rate. Any of the above or any combination thereof, indicates the body is having difficulty dealing with whatever it is handling, and I advise you to take a trip to your health care professional and seek his/her advice.

All in all, fever should be viewed as a good sign as the nervous system and immune system are doing exactly what they are designed to do. I suggest that the next time your child has a fever, understand the reason for the fever, but do not jump the gun and try to lower your child's temperature; you may actually be delaying recovery!

And while we are on the subject of monkeying around with fever, etc., I thought that I would make you aware of a popular cold remedy ingredient which has been linked with strokes in women and seizures in children.

The FDA *recommends* that everyone stop taking anything containing **phenylpropanolamine**. It has been linked to increased hemorrhagic stroke among women ages 18–49 in the three days after starting the use of medication which contains this ingredient. It has also been linked with seizures in children – not a desirable side-effect!

The manufacturer of Triaminic stated they are voluntarily recalling the following medicines (The following are all registered products of individual companies):

- orange 3D cold & allergy
- cherry (pink) 3D cold & cough
- berry 3D cough relief

You may want to be aware that the following medications contain phenylpropanolamine (The following are all registered products of individual companies):

- Acutrim diet gum appetite suppressant plus dietary supplements

- Acutrim maximum strength appetite control
- Alka-Seltzer plus children's cold medicine effervescent
- Alka-Seltzer plus cold & medicine (cherry or orange)
- Alka-Seltzer plus cold & medicine original
- Alka-Seltzer plus cold & flu medicine effervescent
- Alka-Seltzer plus cold & sinus effervescent
- Alka-Seltzer plus night-time cold medicine effervescent
- BC allergy sinus cold powder
- BC sinus cold powder
- Comtrex deep chest cold & congestion relief
- Comtrex flu therapy & fever relief day and night
- Contac 12-hour cold capsules
- Contac 12-hour caplets
- Coricidin D cold, flu & sinus
- Dexatrim caffeine free
- Dexatrim extended duration
- Dexatrim gelcaps
- Dexatrim vitamin C/caffeine free
- Dimetapp cold & allergy chewable tablets
- Dimetapp cold & cough liqui-gels
- Dimetapp DM cold & cough elixir
- Dimetapp elixir
- Dimetapp 4 hour liquid gels
- Dimetapp 4 hour tablets
- Dimetapp 12 hour extentabs
- Naldecon DX pediatric drops
- Permathene mega-16
- Robitussin CF
- Tavist-D 12 hour relief of sinus & nasal congestion
- Triaminic DM cough relief
- Triaminic expectorant chest & head congestion
- Triaminic syrup cold & allergy

I want to stress the point that there is no such thing as a "safe drug" – all have side-effects. The biggest difficulty is that what was considered safe yesterday, may be proven to be fatal tomorrow!

12. Ear Infections

You are suddenly awakened out of a well-deserved sleep. Your child is crying in the next room with sudden and intense pain in her ear. She is flushed, hot, and glassy-eyed with fever. You panic. Childhood ear infections (Otitis Media) are often very frightening to parents mostly because they appear suddenly, usually at night, with little warning.

The most common treatments used for ear infections are antibiotics, decongestants, antipyretics (fever medication), and tympanostomy (tubes in the ears). You may be surprised to learn that the benefits of all of these are highly questionable.

For example, *The Lancet,* a major medical research journal, found that recovery time was about the same for children whether medical intervention happened or nothing was done at all.[45] (I covered a little on this topic in the previous chapter) Another study[46] from the *Archives of Otolaryngology,* showed that "88 percent of children with Otitis Media never needed antibiotics, and antibiotics did not shorten the lifespan of the disease." As a matter of fact, an issue of *Newsweek Magazine* reported that antibiotics are not nearly as effective as the body's own immune system. How about that! What a concept!

For parents frustrated with recurring ear infections, the EENT (ear, eye, nose, and throat) specialist will most likely prescribe the "rite of tympanostomy" – words from the late Dr. Robert Mendelsohn, a friend, and a self- proclaimed "medical heretic." It is a surgical procedure whereby your child is anesthetized so that a tube can be placed in his or her eardrum to drain fluid. Research, however, indicates that this procedure does little to eliminate the problem. It simply reduces pressure and fluid buildup. It is no panacea for ear infections! Parents, however, have been sold on the idea that tubes in the ears are some kind of a cure for ear infections. Most mothers I met in my

---

[45] Van Buchem, F. L., Dunk, J.H.M., Van'thof, M. A., *Therapy of Acute Otitis media: myringonomy, antibiotics or neither?*, Lancet, October 24, 1981, pp. 883-887.

[46] Diamant, M., Diamant, B., *Abuse and timing of use of antibiotics in acute otitis media*, Archives of Otolaryngology, 1074, 226-232.

office, whose children have chronic and recurring ear infections, have already had the "tube thing" done – with no success. This whole concept of surgically placing tubes in the ears of young children to eliminate ear infections is absurd. The middle-ages come to mind!

Whether or not to give a child tympanostomy tubes ... tubes in the ears ... is a debate that has raged in medicine for two decades. One of the major arguments in favor of tubes is that if children have fluid behind the middle ear it can cut down on their ability to hear and can potentially lead to learning problems. But a report in the New England Journal of Medicine says this is not the case. According to the report, in children younger than three years of age who have persistent otitis media, prompt insertion of tympanostomy tubes does not measurably improve developmental outcomes. The procedure has little long-term with respect to hearing behavior or learning development.

Implanting ear tubes, an operation done on hundreds of thousands of toddlers each year, does not appear to improve their speech and learning development and may not be worth the risk and the cost, another study found. Researchers in Pittsburgh looked at two groups of toddlers: those who got ear tubes after three months of fluid in their ears (the standard guideline) and those who waited up to nine months before tubes were inserted. The children were tested for speech, language, learning, and behavior when they turned three. "The bottom line was there wasn't any difference in the development outcomes as best we could measure them at age 3," said Dr. Jack L. Paradise of Children's Hospital of Pittsburgh.

Paradise, however, warned that there is a risk of complications from the anaesthesia. Also, he said, the tubes sometimes leave perforations in the eardrums or scar them, or cause chronic drainage from the ear. "If tubes were absolutely harmless and free, then I think you might say, 'Well, let's have the tubes to be sure'," Paradise said. But tubes themselves carry risk and, of course, there's cost involved. So it becomes a matter of ... which set of risks would you rather take? Paradise said he would hold off inserting tubes if the only concern was developmental problems from hearing loss. There you have it! Yet millions of these operations are performed in Canada and the United

States each year when controlled clinical studies have determined that there was "no benefit gained from the placement of tubes." As a matter of fact, they actually create complications Paradise mentioned – such as scar formation on the eardrum leading to hearing loss. Not a desirable side effect! The biggest problem with these medical treatments is that they attempt to interfere with the body's own healing ability and discount the power of the body to heal. As a result, they don't work!

Let's look at this closely. The Eustachian tube (the small tube which connects the nasal cavity to the inner ear) is at a different angle in children and, therefore, they are prone to infections, at least that is what most parents are told. (If that were the reason for ear infections, then **ALL** children would have ear infections until the tube matured. Most of you have probably noticed that this is not the case.) Other reasons parents are given as to why their children have chronic ear infections include:

- It is a normal part of childhood. Nonsense!

- "Your child has a *tendency* toward ear infections so we'll just put him on a low dose of antibiotics as a preventive measure." (What bunk! I'll tell you what is true. The normal tendency is NOT to have ear infections!)

From my perspective, I see ear infections as a malfunction of the immune system and lowered resistance. In other words, the child's body is not able to fight off or prevent the infection. The main cause of lowered immune resistance in a child is, most often, the process of delivery. Yes, **birth**. It can be very traumatic. The stress of the average, uncomplicated delivery can cause a vertebral subluxation of the delicate segments of a baby's spine, thereby affecting the way a child's nervous system and immune system react to the world around him. In their landmark research studies Dr. Gutman and Dr. Biedermann examined hundreds of newborn infants and concluded that, *"an unhealthy spine at birth causes lowered resistance to infection, especially ear, nose, and throat infection."* [36, 37]

In my own practice, which was largely pediatric, most children I saw with ear infections did have a vertebral subluxation in their spine, affecting the way their nervous system controlled their resistance to infection. By eliminating this subluxation, the child's normal resistance was increased and the threat of ear infection was minimized. You see, it's not a matter of discovering yet another "wonder" antibiotic to drug your child with. It is a matter of having your child's body function better all by itself. What a novel idea!

I remember a public lecture I held at our Centre on the topic of Chronic Ear infections once. Let me tell you this: our lecture theatre was packed with parents – mostly moms. There were also two uninvited guests at the back of the room and these two people attempted to ridicule what I was saying. Finally one of the mothers stood up and asked these two gentlemen to please leave – to the applause of everyone present. I later discovered that my two guests were two EENT specialists – the only two in town. They probably felt threatened by a wellness approach to health care.

As well as chiropractic care, which I feel is essential; you may want to try the following to help your child:

- Vitamin C, 1000-5000 mg daily.
- Echinacea tincture, 20 drops, 2 times per day mixed with a few drops of orange juice for taste. Try for one week and discontinue for one week.
- Zinc lozenges, although kids can't stand these. Use as a last resort.
- Warmed olive oil drops into the affected ear two or three times per day for 2-3 days.

One of my dear patients, Monique, mother of four delightful munchkins, told me of an onion poultice which she has used and which will reduce your child's pain during an episode of an ear infection: *Slice some onions, quick fry in a skillet for a minute only, and place on the affected ear. (Wrap the onions in a cloth first.)* I can just visualize some people not wrapping the onions first. Although I have not attempted this "treatment." Monique swears by it.

* * *

Dear Dr. Ressel,

My son and I have been patients of yours for approximately three months. I originally came to you because my son had been experiencing chronic ear infections In a five-week period of time, he has been diagnosed with four ear infections, and treated with antibiotics three times.

My husband and I had used the services of a different chiropractor a couple of years before, with less than stellar results. I did not realize, at the time, that there are two different approaches to chiropractic. His approach was to treat stiff, sore backs, with no vision as to the Wellness of the individual, whereas your practice concentrated solely on the health and Wellness of the patient.

What really struck me the first time we met was your obvious belief in what you do, and your fire to make me a believer. In theory, what you said made sense to me, but I was still somewhat skeptical. Could subluxations of the spine really be the cause of so many diseases and conditions? Could the "cure" really be as simple as adjusting the spine to make the nervous system function properly?

My son and I started on a course of treatment the following week. He has not had any ear infections since then. One of the more interesting things that you told me during my initial examination was that one of the vertebrae in my neck felt like it might be in the early stages of arthritis and that this region controls thyroid function. The reason I found this so interesting is that three and a half years ago I was diagnosed with Grave's Disease (hyperthyroidism). I began to wonder if what you said might actually be true.

Since the birth of my son, I have seen two massage therapists, a physiotherapist and a chiropractor. None of them had been able to give me any long-term relief, and some of them didn't even give me any short-term relief. After only three months in your care, I must say that I can't remember ever feeling this good.

-Amy Collard

13. Bed Wetting
Nocturnal Enuresis

Wet blankets and sheets in the morning, soaked, smelly pajamas and a very uncomfortable child – this is the picture of bed-wetting (Natural Enuresis) for children.

Enuresis, simply stated, is bed-wetting past the usual time a child is potty trained. It is estimated that one out of five young children wets the bed regularly. This means that 20 percent of five to eight year-olds wet their bed – not OK. Imagine what this does to a child's self esteem. Incidentally, the oldest patient I have seen with this condition was a 21-year-old dental hygienist – imagine how she must have felt!

Over time, various reasons have been proposed as the cause of bed- wetting such as psychological, habitual, etc. Many methods have been used to "treat" this affliction; alarm systems in the bed, electric shocks, hypnosis, drugs, waking the child, psychotherapy, etc. None of these have had much of an affect.

Bed-wetting occurs when there is improper function of the nerves, which control the flow of urine from the bladder and regulate the function of the bladder sphincter, or valve. One of these nerves is under voluntary control, which means you go when you want to. The other is on "autopilot" or "automatic." In other words, the child has no voluntary control over this particular one. The function of these two nerves is controlled by the child's nervous system, which keeps both in check and balance. Beware of ads suggesting that it is OK for children to wet the bed because now there are school age diapers available. These ads seem to suggest that some children's bladders may not have developed properly and so a diaper is the answer. Nonsense! This is called marketing!

I mentioned this issue earlier; have you noticed ads recently, mentioning a new "disease?" I have. Medicine and the pharmaceutical industry have developed a new disease. It is called the "**Overactive Bladder Disease.**" And as you may have guessed, there is a drug to deal with the condition.

The same holds true for adult diapers – "Depends" or "Attends." Instead of dealing with the reason WHY the bladder is not functioning, it is much more profitable to put adults and school age children in "diapers." Marketing states that it is now socially acceptable to go shopping and do your business as you walk because you are wearing diapers.

I'll let you draw your own conclusions.

Early in my practice I found, as do most chiropractors treating children that those who are bedwetters respond very well to chiropractic care. The reason for this is quite simple. We deal with removing any interference to the normal function of the nervous system. Throughout this book I have explained our health approach, where we apply this concept to a child whose nervous system control of his or her bladder is lacking. The results are actually quite amazing. If your child is experiencing difficulty, I urge you to talk to a family chiropractor as soon as possible.

* * *

Michael's Story.

In December of 1997, about one and half weeks before school was out for Christmas break, I noticed that Michael was starting to come home from school with "wet" pants. This was quite unusual for him, as he has never had a problem with incontinence or bed-wetting. My first thought was that something might have been bothering him at school but after talking to him, it seemed to be that things were okay. The week before Christmas break, the incontinence continued but he woke up one morning and said that his legs hurt. I didn't think that was anything to worry about, perhaps just "growing pains." A couple of days later, he woke up complaining about his feet hurting. Again, I didn't know what to make of this, if anything, but both my husband and I were getting frustrated with the incontinence. We thought that he was just being "lazy" and more concerned with playing than taking the time to go to the bathroom. On the last day of school, he woke up and said that his hips hurt, and he was sort of limping a little. I told him that I would keep an eye on him today and check up on him at the school later that morning. As I walked Michael to the bus stop that morning. I noticed that he really was limping. I called him over to me and hugged him and he said he was telling the truth. At that point I got a lump in my throat and was choked up, because I could see that he was somewhat worried. He chose to get on the bus and I told him if he needed to tell the teacher to call me and pick him up.

By the time I got to the school at about 11:45, his teacher spotted me outside the classroom and came out to talk to me. She had noticed that he was limping in gym class that morning. He had found it difficult to participate and sat it out. She was quite concerned, as was I, at that point. It made no sense to me. I called Michael out of the classroom and asked him how he was feeling. He was definitely not himself. He had pain in his hips and was limping, but at this point he didn't want to leave, because like any normal child, he didn't want to miss the class Christmas party. I told him that if he got worse to have the teacher call me right away. I picked him up a little early at the end of the day and brought him to a pediatric walk-in clinic.

When we went into the exam room, Michael's pants were wet, and I explained this to the doctor along with his other symptoms. The doctor examined him and sent us to the lab for a urine culture. She said she thought it was probably a urinary tract infection, and wanted him to get started on an antibiotic right away. When we got home, I immediately started him on the antibiotics. At this point, his limp had gotten worse.

On Saturday morning, he woke up and he was very unstable on his feet. That night, my husband had to work a midnight shift and I was very worried so I put Michael in my bed to keep a close eye on him. During the day he had started complaining that his feet were itchy. I lay beside him that night, and noticed that his legs from the knee down were very cold and half-dozed, and he kept asking in a sort of cry for me to scratch them continually. So I did but as time went on, he was very restless, and the itchiness was driving him crazy. He was moaning and uttering words in his sleep and I didn't know what was happening. It almost seemed like he was hallucinating. I was very scared. I thought he might have been having a reaction to the antibiotic so I called my neighbour to stay with the girls around 2:00 a.m. while I took him to the hospital. At this point, Michael could no longer stand. I had to carry him into the car and use the wheelchair at the hospital.

The emergency room doctor examined him. Michael was trickling urine at this point. I told the doctor that we had been at the clinic on Friday afternoon and that he was on antibiotics for a probable urinary tract infection. This doctor did a quick urine test as well and the results came back negative, so there was nothing further he could do. I asked if the antibiotics could have cleared an infection that quickly and he said that it was highly unlikely. To make sure, I called for the results of the original urine culture done on the Friday. Again, I questioned why would he be in such pain and unable to walk if there was nothing wrong. The doctor had the nurse give Michael some Tylenol and we went home.

Early Monday morning I called for the urine test results. They came back negative. I then called Michael's doctor who advised I bring him in right away. At this point Michael was unable to pass urine. His doctor noted that his bladder was distended almost to his navel and said that he would require a catheter. After an extensive exam, his doctor explained that he thought it might be Guillain Barre Syndrome and sent me to the hospital for another opinion from another pediatrician. At the hospital, he was immediately catheterized. The pediatrician did her examination and sent Michael for a spinal x-ray. By this time, mid-afternoon, Michael had no feeling in his legs, they were very cold and he was in pain. This doctor had noted that among these other symptoms his anal opening was enlarged; she feared a spinal tumour. After explaining her findings and that she needed to rule this out, she proceeded to make arrangements to have Michael ambulanced to Sick Kids Hospital that evening.

Once we arrived at the hospital, there was a team of doctors who conducted their own examinations. I had been asked about any symptoms, falls, etc. Michael had not been sick in the recent past. I did recall a fall he had about a month previous and told them about it. Michael had slid down a flight of carpeted stairs on his bottom and I remembered it because when he got to the bottom, he was crying and told me that it "really hurt." He seemed to be fine after that and I didn't think about it until this happened. He was then taken for a MRI. We were told that if it was a tumour of this sort, they would operate immediately and they were prepared for it. They had plenty of his blood type on hand and would proceed quickly as they said that time was crucial at this point. There was no time to waste.

We went for a MRI, but after several hours of attempting this, we had to stop. Michael was in pain and very frightened and could not stay still. Although my husband and I were at his feet, reaching in to touch him throughout the whole time, reassuring him, it wouldn't work. He was petrified of the sounds and scared about what was happening to him. They stopped at midnight and said we would try again first thing in the morning. About one o'clock that morning, a nurse came in to start an IV and started Michael on a strong dosage of Decadron. The doctor explained the urgency in administering the corticosteroid A.S.A.P., and so it was done.

By 8:00 a.m. Tuesday morning, Michael was back for the MRI. They put him out with anesthetic and taken in. We had also been asked to give consent to a spinal tap. At this point we were told that Michael would go straight to surgery after the MRI was done because again, they needed to act quickly. Words could never describe the despair and fear that were going through us while Michael was in. I cried and prayed and cried and prayed as my husband sat beside me trying to keep himself together while comforting me. My emotions were uncontrollable, I couldn't believe how quickly everything was happening and we had no control over any of this.

A while later, a doctor came out and by some miracle, explained that they would not be operating on Michael, and that it did not appear to be a tumour. We would be spoken to later by his doctor – but I knew that this was our first blessing!

Michael continued with the Decadron Ranitidine for his stomach and an antibiotic to prevent infection from the catheterization. The doctor had Michael's catheter removed to reduce the risk of infection so Michael had to be catheterized every four to six hours. It took two to three nurses and me by his side each time this had to be done. He was horrified by the whole experience each time, and so was I. Michael was bedridden, very fragile, and it was painful for him to move at all. It was either that day or on the Wednesday that all of a sudden Michael was overcome with pain for about ten minutes. I didn't know what to do, I couldn't move him at all and he was screaming. I tried to comfort him as best as I could, and shortly after, I realized that he had a bowel movement. The pressure of his waste trying to pass through had caused the pain, and he couldn't feel what was happening. After that time, I knew the signs when it was going to happen, and just tried to relax and distract him as much as possible.

Being that it was during the Christmas holidays, there were always many new doctors that were coming in. We asked daily, but they didn't have any answers. We were just told that they were ruling out things. The numbness in the legs continued, and he continued to experience pain as well as the visible side effects of the drugs. An abdominal ultrasound was done, as well as nerve conduction studies. All came back normal. We were told the protein levels in his spinal fluid were normal. Michael was experiencing some chest pain making it difficult to breathe at one point and they did an ECG; all was okay. I used a saline bag, warmed it up in the microwave and placed in the chest area to try to relax him.

Emotionally, Michael was very angry and depressed. Although he was very cooperative with all his doctors and nurses it was when he was with mom and dad that he let his anger out. It was very draining but we knew we had to be strong and deal with it as best as we could.

On Christmas Day, a nurse came in and gave him a bath, which was uncomfortable for him because sitting up caused pain. She put him upright in a wheelchair and I wheeled him through the halls. About an hour later, I noticed that Michael had somehow moved his body and he was more on his side. We were both ecstatic about this and by the time our family came to the hospital later that day he was moving about in his wheelchair with more ease. From Christmas day, he started to show more signs of improvement with respect to his mobility, and then he slowly started to regain some feeling back in his feet and legs. Michael was in physiotherapy as well. He was given Decadron for one week and then changed to Prednisone. Michael's recovery was quite remarkable. Just after Christmas, Michael was given a walker and we would try to walk for a bit every few hours. A couple of days later, he had a rollator. On New Year's Eve day, Michael was given a bicycle to ride in the hallways (I thought they were joking). Well everyone was amazed with Michael on his bicycle. He was very happy to ride his bike.

On New Year's Eve, we had arranged for a hospital pass for a few hours to have dinner with family we had in Toronto. As they had three children, we thought it would be great "spiritual"' medicine. I had been trying to get Michael to urinate on his own to see if he might have regained that function too. He had to be catheterized before we left, so I had Michael try on his own first. He pushed and pushed and for the first time, he did it! He was very happy, especially since he didn't have to be catheterized for this time. We left on our pass, and as I thought, it was just what he needed. He was smiling, laughing and just being a boy among the other kids. That night, he surprised me by coming upstairs. He did a flight of steps, one by one with assistance. Later that evening, he was able to urinate again on his own. He was very encouraged by this.

Michael was discharged on January 2nd. His diagnosis (through process of elimination) was Acute Transverse Myelitis (lower spinal cord, mostly T2). His condition upon discharge was mild weakness (4+/5) of hip extensors and abductors and foot flexors/extensors. Michael was on a timed void until he regained full function (if he did). He was to be weaned off the Prednisone over the next 10 days and arrangements for continued physiotherapy were made in our hometown. By the end of January, Michael had completed his physiotherapy.

A follow up was done at the hospital one month later, where it was noted that the Transverse Myelitis was resolved. Another follow up was scheduled for six months time which was in August, 1998. Neurologically, Michael was found to be normal and I discussed with the doctor the problems with Michael's incontinence. His recommendation was to see a pediatric urologist and have the bladder tested (VCUG).

Once I returned home from his hospital stay, I immediately began to research Transverse Myelitis. Both my husband and I accepted the diagnosis we were given but were uncomfortable with it. Although Michael's situation has similarities to TM, I read case upon case which had very different outcomes to Michael's. I became a member of the TM Association support group and was in contact with others who had TM. If he truly did have TM, we're very fortunate for the recovery he made as most don't make such a recovery.

From the time Michael came home, to this day, we have been dealing with incontinence. He has been trying to adhere to the "timed void" however, being a third grade 8-year-old, he'd rather not be "different," or want to "miss out" on what the other kids are doing, therefore, he doesn't always make it his first priority. In the spring of 1998, Michael had urinary tract infections several times so to prevent further infections and possible damage to the kidneys, he was put on an antibiotic (low maintenance dose.) He's had tests done to determine whether the kidneys had been affected, and fortunately they have not. In as much as we didn't want him to be taking an antibiotic daily, for the next year, we felt we had no choice. It seemed that the measures I had taken to prevent these infections weren't working.

During the next year, I could see the incontinence seemed to have become a daily thing. Our frustration as parents was getting worse, because we didn't see any improvements. The doctor said he couldn't do anything and that we had to let time takes its course. I would not subject him to any more invasive procedures just so we could confirm that he had a problem, nor did we want to treat his bladder with any more drugs that would have horrible side effects.

It was in December of 1998, when I first had the privilege to meet Dr. Ressel, who had briefly been told of Michael's situation by my brother. I attended a seminar given by Dr. Ressel, and afterwards, spoke briefly to him about the situation. He wasted no time and saw Michael within two days. When we met again for the report of his findings, both my husband and I were shocked at what he had to say, because it made SENSE and was LOGICAL!

Dr. Ressel determined that the incident with the staircase caused a vertebral subluxation. This evoked the normal tissue inflammatory response, which produced neurologic malfunction. The manifestations were clear: loss of rectal tone, bladder and bowel incontinence, excessive gastrointestinal gas, loss of ambulatory function, paresthesias, sensory changes and vasoconstriction in the lower limbs. Michael had health challenges preceding the staircase incident. His APGAR score depicted a fairly difficult birth, which produced a subluxation that in turn, changed the normal architecture of his spine. With this said, we are now working on restoring Michael back to optimum health, it may take time, but at least we know what we're dealing with.

-Aggie and Joe Agnino

14. Asthma

Most likely someone you know is suffering with this condition. Could be your child, a parent, someone close to you, or even yourself. I say this because there are thousands of North American children (and adults) afflicted with difficulty of breathing.

A report on the status of asthma in the United States conducted by the Pew Environmental Commission, estimates Asthma cases will double by the year 2020. That means that one out of every 14 people will suffer from this condition. Currently, Asthma costs $11 billion annually and it is the number one reason for school absenteeism. It accounts for almost two million hospital visits and 5000 deaths yearly in the United States. From 1980 to 1994 the overall number of Asthma sufferers increased by 75 percent and 160 percent specifically in youngsters under four. The Department of Health and Human Services (Healthy People 2000 Initiative) includes an Asthma strategy, although this report[47] states, "it will not be effective in reversing this alarming trend." A review of the 1999 HHS research budget revealed that 70 percent of the funds designated for Asthma were spent on treatment and drug research while less than nine percent was targeted for prevention.

"Almost nothing is going towards tracking the disease and very little is going towards prevention and discovering the cause of the disease," states Dr. Paul Lock, Deputy Commissioner of the commission on May 17, 2000.[48]

It is estimated that in the next twenty-five years, 50 percent of all children will have difficulty in catching their breath – Not OK! Why is this "*dis* ease" becoming so rampant? United Kingdom scientists are beginning a hospital trial to see the affects of certain bacteria on Asthma. "There is a global network of biological asthma research which has demonstrated that the lower the exposure of a baby to certain types of bacteria, the higher the risk of Asthma," states Dr. Charles Warner, child coordinator and professor of child's health at the University of South Hampton.

---

[47] *Healthy People 2000*, National Health Promotion and Disease Prevention Objectives, Conference edition: Summary US Department of Health and Human Services, Public Health Service.

[48] PEW Environmental Health Commission, John Hopkins School of Public Health, Reuters Health, May 17, 2000.

I mentioned this tid-bit earlier; researchers are going to add a low dose of bacteria, which is commonly found in dirt (*please refer to my "DIRT" chapter*) to 400 babies' diet, whose families have a history of Asthma. They will then study and assess the child's risk of developing asthma. It is hoped that the bacteria will eventually play a role in boosting the children's immune system. Consumers have been driven to be afraid of bacteria, fostering an inappropriate use of antibiotics ("just-in-case" prescriptions), and a market saturated with antibacterial soaps and cleaners. Not only have we created an environment in which resistant super-bug bacteria can thrive, but we also kill bacteria, which are actually beneficial and essential to balance the internal environment of our bodies.

Let's look at this closer.

Breathing is a process whereby your body takes air from the outside. This air then passes through your nose, windpipe, and your bronchi. These are all parts of your "air conditioning" system, so to speak. This air is then filtered, purified, cleansed, warmed, and humidified before it enters your lungs. Think about the science behind this for a moment. There are amazing biofeedback loops at work here that inform your brain whether the air you are breathing in is too cold, too dry, too polluted, etc. These messages are relayed to your brain, which then makes minute corrections to your 'program' every second that you are alive. It is an amazing process and happens very exactly under the perfect guidance of your nervous system. Yes, your nervous system is responsible for this function.

So, what then is Asthma?

In children (and adults) who have Asthma, the small tubes in the lungs, called bronchioles, become inflamed and irritated. They then contract and even spasm and produce mucous, which tend to plug up the breathing passages. Children can literally gasp for air. These "attacks" can last minutes or hours and can persist for a lifetime.

It is generally felt that an Asthma attack can be triggered by allergies, stress, pollen, pollution, etc. It can be life threatening. These children are condemned to a life of bronchodilators, drugs, and cortisone, all of which have serious side effects. These side effects can be either immediate or develop over a lifetime of chronic drug use. Asthma is said to be the leading cause of chronic illness among children. Not a fun thing to have. It is definitely a condition best avoided.

Here is the catch however: Have you ever wondered why some children subjected to the same stresses, pollens, etc., develop Asthma while others do not? After all, if Asthma were caused by all the factors the public has been led to believe, then all children would have it. Right? Wrong! Only some do, and their numbers have been rising steadily.

Why (my favourite question)? The standard medical first-line approach to clearing Asthma is to prescribe inhalant steroids. These often reduce the frequency and intensity of Asthma attacks, but not without a price. Steroid use has been linked to osteoporosis, stunted growth in children and cataracts. The effects of long-term use are unknown since these drugs are so new. Steroids substitute for and decrease the body's ability to make its own steroids, and to respond to stress as well as suppressing the immune system. Those taking high doses of these drugs are warned to avoid vaccinations that are made up of live viruses (MMR, Polio, Chicken Pox). If any of these viruses are contacted while steroids are being used, it could be life threatening. Although these drugs are often taken by pregnant and breast-feeding mothers they have not been tested for safety under these instances (though it stands to reason that these drugs will have similar effects on babies).

As I mentioned earlier, all drugs cross the placental barrier and affect the baby. According to a recent study, "the majority of adults and children with asthma experience unwanted side affects of medication; such as feeling generally restless, shaky hands, shaky feet, racing heartbeat, etc. These side effects have prompted 1 in 3 adults to reduce their medication and cause one in four to skip a dose at some point."

Some authorities feel that asthma is really a reaction to a lack of proper hydration of the body; that it is a lack of water. They, therefore, suggest drinking plenty of *pure* water to hydrate the body. In my practice, I have not met many children who like to drink pure water; it is boring. If you believe this is the solution, then I recommend that you use a fruit concentrate, such as *Ribena Blackcurrant Concentrate*, mixed with 5 parts water for taste. It is an English drink but moms can pick it up in most grocery stores.

Many researchers, on the other hand, have found that asthma seems to be related to our current vaccination program. There are increasing numbers of scientists and practitioners who support this conclusion. Bart Classen M.D., of Classen Immunotherapies in Maryland, is among the most vociferous. (You are welcome to visit his web site at *www.vaccines.net.*)

Vaccination alters the normal immune response and makes a child's immune system overreact to something perfectly innocuous. (I will be discussing vaccination and its effects on the health of our children later). As a result, a child's immune system is over-stimulated and becomes over-sensitive. Air, for example, that would not bother a normal person, has an adverse effect of a child whose nervous and immune systems are "overloaded."

D. D. Palmer, the discoverer of chiropractic, once said it this way, "I desired to know why one person was ailing and his associate, eating at the same table, working in the same shop, was not. Why? What differences were in the two persons that caused one to have Asthma while his partner escaped? Why?"

Doctors of Chiropractic have been helping children with asthma for years. I have had the good fortune of being able to have helped hundreds of children with this condition. How does Chiropractic relate to Asthma you ask? Remember I mentioned that the body is a self-healing, self-regulating organism? Also, remember that the nervous system is the central computer that runs the whole body and all of its functions; the function of the arms, legs, digestive system, sinuses, your immune system, and even the lungs and bronchioles. Every part of your being is under the control of your nervous system. It is your very own Internet.

As long as the nervous system is allowed to function with no interference, the body should function normally. Often, however, some of the vertebrae of the spine become subluxated, affecting the way the nervous system controls body functions. Chiropractors call this *malfunction*. It simply means that the body is no longer performing according to the program; it is no longer working normally. By correcting these subluxations, chiropractors eliminate interference to the nervous system allowing normal function. By eliminating interference to the nervous system, we can help the body work normally again. With no drugs! I like that.

As well as chiropractic care, which is essential, there are a number of natural supplements you can obtain from a health food store to help yourself and your child through a trying period.

- **Vitamin B complex plus C -** It stimulates the immune system, and reduces the effects of stress.

- **Quercetin with Bromelain -** These together act as an immuno-stimulant and antiinflammatory agent.

- **Vitamin A -** This is beneficial for tissue repairs.

- **Lobelia -** Helpful during an attack. It is an expectorant and relaxes the muscle walls of the bronchial tree

- **Coenzyme Q10 -** This helps to counteract the release of histamine, which induces local tissue swelling.

- **Magnesium and calcium -** Tend to cause some dilation of the muscle walls of the bronchi.

Some authorities suggest bee pollen or propolis. I have found that such bee products often cause allergic reactions in children, and I feel they should be avoided.

* * *

Dear Dr. Ressel,

Our eldest daughter, Clarisse, then aged six, was continually being diagnosed with bronchitis and has much difficulty breathing on a good day. My husband was diagnosed with asthma as a child, and this was being considered for Clarisse as well. "Let's just give this a try and see what happens" assured the doctor on call at a walk-in medical clinic, as she handed me the prescription for puffers. I wasn't comfortable with the solution; something in my gut told me there had to be another way. But I also told myself that this was the third time this term that Clarisse had to stay home from school for a week to recuperate. I spoke to her teacher about this final episode, and told her I wished I could find an answer other than drugs. She thought that it was worth a try to see Dr. Ogi Ressel and told me that another family at the school had good results from him for their children's various ailments. I decided to speak with this other mother and I still remember her words, "My children haven't gone to see a medical doctor in two years and we haven't had to fill a prescription ever since." It sounded very encouraging.

I spoke with my husband about it and we decided to give Dr. Ressel a call. During our initial appointment he explained to us how the spinal column worked and how the nervous system reached out to every organ and every corner of our body through the spine. When the vertebrae was subluxated, the power to the various parts of the body was affected thus causing either chronic pain or illness. Through chiropractic care, we could expect to eliminate the subluxations, put the power back into our nervous system, and, therefore, be on the road to Wellness without the use of drugs. So far everything he was saying made a lot of sense. We all, that is to say, my whole family including my husband David, our daughter Clarisse, our four-year old daughter Savannah, our eighteen-month-old Santino and I, were put on individualized programs to achieve Wellness.

That was a year and a half ago. Here are just a few of the ways in which chiropractic care has made out lives better. My husband, after thirty years, has not needed to use his puffers. He hasn't changed anything else about his lifestyle, which includes working sixty-hour weeks and doing cardio and weight bearing workouts several times a week. He feels very good about this new-found freedom.

Clarisse never had to use her puffers and has never experienced another bronchial infection since we've started care. She can now run up and down the soccer field and is the top scoring player on her team. As a matter of fact, none of our children have experienced anything that required taking any prescription drugs, including children's Tylenol. I was pregnant at the time of out first meeting, and I remember thinking back now that it was my easiest pregnancy. I had excruciating pain in my pelvic area with my previous pregnancy and was put on muscle relaxants and told it wouldn't affect my baby – who really wants to take drugs when they're pregnant? So I just put up with the pain and trashed my prescription. Now I wonder why my doctor didn't recommend chiropractic care instead.

Our daughter Paloma was born at home with the assistance of a midwife. I experienced very little back pain and no pain at all between my contractions. She was born without the use of drugs. Paloma began to receive chiropractic care as of her third day of life and we made an informed decision not to immunize her as we were well aware that her "power had been on" since birth. I will admit, however, that I was a bit reluctant to sit through her first major fever and do nothing. I nervously called Dr. Ressel's answering service when her fever hit 104 degrees F. It was 2:00 A.M. Within five minutes Dr. Rudy, another chiropractor at the Centre, called me back and listened to my concerns and made some very insightful comments about the benefits of fever. It's one thing to hear about the usefulness of fever but it's a whole other thing watching your six-month-old baby breathing rapidly and looking comatose. I remember thinking "we've trusted these people this far and there is no reason why we shouldn't trust them now." We let the fever do its job and it broke the next morning all by itself, as they told me it would!

We've gone through colds, the flu, skin disorders, constipation, severe diarrhea, enuresis, mastitis, and the biggest, nastiest headaches that you can ever imagine without so much as an aspirin following our own prescription for Wellness prescribed by none other that our trusted friend,

Dr. Ogi Ressel. From the bottom of our hearts, we would like to thank "Dr. Ogi" and his amazing staff for always being there for us and for showing us the real meaning of being "well-adjusted."

-Monique Philippe, on the behalf of the Philippe/Tonigussi family.

Dear Dr. Ressel,

Before I started to go to a chiropractor I had asthma everyday without doing anything. When I jogged for five minutes I needed my puffer - it was so hard to breathe. When I woke up every morning I got asthma but now it's slowly going away because I visit the chiropractor's place. Dr. Ressel usually adjusts me, but on the odd occasion when he's not there Dr. Rudy adjusts me. I've been going to chiropractor for about four months and I am feeling great.

-Gregory Lis (age 13)

Dear Dr. Ressel,

Before I started going to a chiropractor, I had asthma everyday and had to take a puffer constantly because I would not be able to sleep at night. Then I decided to go to you and I didn't think it would work because nothing has worked before to cure my asthma. But soon after a few adjustments I saw an improvement. Before when I ran around and played sports, I always got asthma and could barely play. Fortunately though, it now is better. After a couple of weeks I only had it in the morning and still sometimes when I ran around. After the first exam when I started going three times a week instead of five, I suddenly started getting asthma some more but soon it stopped and I only had it occasionally in the morning. From then on I had little asthma and sometimes more than normal. But now I rarely have it, except sometimes when I run a lot but that's rare. I have only used my puffer once or twice since I started care. Chiropractic has helped me a lot and I hope it will totally 100 percent take care of my asthma.

-Jacob Lis (age 15)

15. Allergies

Many people feel that when it comes to allergies it is OK to have them. Most feel that it is quite normal to be allergic. Because many other people are also afflicted, there is a sense that somehow there is strength in numbers. That it is OK to have a season for coughing, blowing, wheezing, and sneezing. Or is it?

Thousands of children (and their parents) in communities all over seem to be affected by this allergy thing. For those of you who do not suffer from allergies, you are looked upon with envy during certain times of the year. As you probably already guessed, millions of hard-earned dollars are spent on over-the-counter drugs, weekly shots, and physician visits. Then, there is time-missed from school (or work), and the effect of little "Miss Sneezy" on the family. The toll from allergies is immense.

Why is that? What is it that makes one child allergic and another not? Why would one child be allergic to cats, dogs, fur, feathers, grasses, tree pollens, and my all-time favourite, peanut butter? After all, we all live on the same planet! What is the difference between one individual and another? Aren't we all essentially the same?

If I took one individual with allergies and one without, then boiled them down to their essentials, (if that was possible), I would end up with approximately seventy pounds of chemicals. The rest would be water. The chemical composition would be the same in both individuals. So then, why would one have allergies and the other not, if both were the same?

The comparison is most often seen in how differently each child's body is able to adapt. Very simply put, an allergy is the in- ability of your child's body to handle something which is in their immediate environment: Pollen from trees, from grasses, flowers, peanuts, etc. (There are also allergies to drugs, harsh detergents, and other chemical agents. These allergies are seen as a protective reaction and are not the type I am discussing.) In other words, your child seems to be very sensitive to the pollen, dust, etc., in their immediate environment. This is called being *hypersensitive.*

Think about this for a moment. Something is making your child's body hypersensitive to a perfectly normal part of the environment! Is the solution to eliminate of all the flowers, trees, grasses, etc.? Or does it make more sense to make your child's body function normally, to effectively cope with its environment?

As I discussed earlier, the thing that runs your child's body in a perfect manner, is the nervous system. As long as it is able to control all functions of the body with *no interference*, your child should have the best health possible. If, however, there is interference to the normal function of the nervous system, your child's body will not function properly, and will react poorly to pollens, peanuts, and his/her environment. Chiropractors call this interference a vertebral subluxation. It can be a serious health hazard! By correcting these vertebral subluxations, your child will have a better chance to successfully deal with allergies.

I suggest that if you or your child are somehow mysteriously "afflicted" with allergies, a trip to your family chiropractor should be top on your list of priorities.

16. Scoliosis

"As the twig is bent, so grows the tree." Alexander Pope

Your child has just come home from school with a note from the public health nurse stating that he/she may have scoliosis. The recommendation is that he/she be checked further. Your initial reaction is one of panic, followed by a good measure of guilt. After all, you should have noticed this first; you are the parent! This seems to be a very common scenario - with most parents being unfamiliar with what scoliosis is, how to detect it in their children or what to do about it.

Scoliosis is, very simply, a curvature of the spine. When examined from the back, the spine in scoliosis is bent latterly (sideways) compared to a normal spine which should be straight.

Scoliosis can damage a child's health in a number of ways. In advanced cases, scoliosis tends to place pressure on the heart and lungs. It can also lead to the development of advanced arthritis in the areas of the spine under maximum stress. Posture can be affected. Clothing does not hang properly which can lead to a problem with your child's self-esteem. Athletic ability can be compromised as well. Other complications of scoliosis are too numerous to mention; ultimately, it is a situation that is best avoided.

Most medical literature has placed scoliosis in an 80/20 split between girls and boys respectively. I have had an extensive research paper published in October, 2004, and in it I discussed the issue of Scoliosis is considerable detail.[49] One of the things I have noticed is that the percentage of Scoliosis is roughly at 50 percent between boys and girls – totally different than what is medically accepted. What a surprise!

There are essentially two types of scoliosis:

Fixed – This form is caused primarily by certain genetic malformations of the spine and is very rigid.

---

[49] Ressel Ogi, Rudy Robert, "Vertebral Subluxation Correlated with Somatic, Viceral and Immune Complaints: An Analysis of 650 Children Under Chiropractic Care," JVSR, Oct 18, 2004.

In other words, a child with this type of curvature always has it, no matter what position he or she tends to assume. Although very difficult to deal with, this type is also very rare. This is a good thing.

Functional – This form is by far the most common. This type of curvature can unwind or straighten when a child is in certain positions or postures. Family doctors and/ or specialists most often label it "idiopathic," which means no known cause. (As a side note, I always smirk when hearing these words as I can't help but think of the "pathetic idiots" who have come up with that phraseology. For some reason, they forgot to understand that there is *always* a reason for scoliosis – even if they don't know what it is.)

Historically, medicine has always adopted a "wait and see" attitude towards scoliosis, much to the frustration of parents and children alike. Over the years, there have been a number of breakthroughs, but they have all been proven unsuccessful; body casts, corsets, physiotherapy, etc. Even Dr. Bobechko's muscle stimulator implants of the late 1970s have all proved relatively dismal. Those curvatures which progressed rapidly were eventually scheduled for spinal surgery, where any number of steel Harrington rods were screwed into the spine in the hope of straightening it – a barbaric ritual.

As parents, we must be aware that scoliosis does have a cause. It does not just descend upon a child out of the blue. It will eventually cause other postural changes to which parents will respond in a predictable manner. "Stand up straighter, pull your shoulders back, hold your chin up." These strange postures children assume are not done on purpose to annoy parents. No! The child is not likely even aware of the problem.

A child's development of upright posture; walking, sitting and other complex movements, is a critical period of time. The young developing nervous system often assimilates, differentiates, and adapts to internal and external signals and data. By these processes, this young nervous system actually learns new postural patterns, future habits and reactions, by responding to repetitive and continuous stimuli. Such a developing nervous system is not always able to distinguish between proper and improper data, and so it responds to both. The response of this young nervous system is, again, neither "good nor bad," but rather adaptive to the data that it is continuously being fed, thus being conditioned for future response.

This process of "neurological learning" or "programming" of the nervous system with respect to movement, posture and body function starts a few short months after birth and continues through to preteen years and adolescence.[50] What this means is that the nervous system causes some of the muscles of the spine to become tight and others to relax. This simple example will tend to produce a curvature of the spine. If the nervous system produces a different command, a different form of adaptation will take place. I see this as learned response – a habit.

Dr. Fred Barge, past president of the International Chiropractors Association, wrote a terrific book on Scoliosis.[51] He attributes these phenomena to vertebral subluxation; in other words, interference with the "information highway" affecting the way the nervous systems transmits and processes information about its internal and external environment. I very much agree. These subluxations cause the input data flowing to a child's nervous system to be erroneous. The nervous system responds to this faulty input by abnormal muscle function, thereby producing a curvature of a spine as a means of best dealing with the data. So you see, scoliosis is rarely the problem, it is most often simply the result of a long-standing vertebral subluxation the nervous system is attempting to adapt and handle.

The possibility and number of effects upon normal development by improper nervous system stimuli are vast and far-reaching. Scoliosis is only one such result. In the care of children, a chiropractor's main concern lies with the chronic faulty data that disturbs normal nervous system function. It then becomes of paramount importance to prevent and eliminate this faulty programming before improper and inefficient habits are learned.

---

[50] Ressel, O., *Chiropractic and Children: A Rationale for Care*, ICA Review, 1986.
[51] Barge, F., *Idiopathic Scolosis: Identifiable Causes, Detection and Correction*, Baldwin Brothers, Inc., second edition 1986.

As you know by now, I see vertebral subluxations as a major threat to a child's health and well-being. I also feel that all children should be checked by a chiropractor as soon as possible to detect the presence of any vertebral subluxations. I am including a posture chart, which will make it easier for you, as parents, to do a scoliosis and posture test at home. Here are the instructions. They are actually quite simple.

POSTURAL ASSESSMENT

How do your children stack up?

1. Have your child stand still (that may be a feat in itself), with his or her back to you.
2. Match the posture of the various body areas on the chart to the posture your child has assumed and place your score on the right side of the form. Postural deviations usually indicate an underlying problem. Add up the score. Ideally, it should not be over five. If it is, then your child may be developing scoliosis. I suggest that a chiropractic consultation would be in order.

17. Growing Pains

Have you ever experienced the heartbreak of having your child cry at bedtime with what seems to be to indescribable pains in his/ her legs? You may have tried all the standard parent remedies such as walking, reading, hot towels, cuddling, massaging the legs, all to no avail. The pains still persist. Eventually your child finally falls asleep from sheer exhaustion, and you simply dread a repeat performance the next day. Your heartstrings and nerves have had it. Finally, out of pure frustration you seek professional help only to be told that it is simply "growing pains," and are told that, "your child will eventually grow out of it." Concerned parents often hear such puzzling comments. What is worse is that they may actually believe them.

You were probably told that your child's legs hurt because the bones, ligaments and muscles are developing and stretching and a little pain is a normal part of the process. Apparently all these tissues and bones all grow differently and *should* cause pain. This has always been traditionally explained as a normal part of childhood. Many concerned parents have believed this theory for years, because at first glance, it seems fairly sound. It appears to be plausible and after all, parents are not trained as doctors.

But think about this just for a moment.

When did it ever hurt to grow? And why only the legs? Don't the arms grow? What about the nose, the fingers, and all the other parts of body? Why don't they hurt? You are suddenly beginning to see that the explanations most parents hear are not only untrue but also illogical.

If that's the case then, what is the real reason of these pains? Let's look at this with a magnifying glass.

Growing pains are defined as pains in the limbs and joints of children often attributed to rapid growth. It is a mistake, however, to attribute any pain to growing. Growth is a natural process occurring in the body that increases size with gradual addition or infusion of materials. The human body is complex in its development and growth, but it is a positive not painful process.

Growth occurs very rapidly during early infancy. Middle infancy is marked by gain of control over large muscle groups. Between the ages of two and one-half to eleven years, physiological growth rates actually lessen. Since a child's height and weight then changes slowly, he/she is able to gain bigger and better balance in his/her sensor-motor operations during this period of development.

The next stage of development is puberty and usually occurs between the ages of ten and fifteen. This stage of rapid growth and maturation is most often associated with the term "growing pains." Rapid growth starts with a release of new genetic information by certain "organizing" cells. This information activates the endocrine system and the glands of that system then produce hormones, which will activate growth. The pituitary glands actually secrete several hormones directly related to growth. Somatotrophin controls the size of the individual, especially the length of the limbs. The thyroid gland secretes Thyroxine, which greatly influences the metabolism of the body. These hormones, acting together, activate the cells of the body to increase and promote rapid growth.

The maturation of the skeleton is a near perfect example of growth engineering. Molding itself as it grows, it adapts to its own growth. The vertebral column requires two more curves than it had at birth and the legs become proportionately longer with the trunk shorter. While bone development is consistent with the general rate of physical maturation, the speed of muscular growth is influenced by the amount of physical exercise.

Muscles lengthen proportionately to bone growth and so do the ligaments attached to these bones. In other words, everything grows at a normal, perfect rate – no pain! But for muscles to increase in size, physical exercise is needed – and at that age children are generally very active.

Even their everyday activities promote a certain degree of muscular development. The children that are super active will increase more, but not until the late stages of puberty are the muscles ready for major development. If major muscle growth should precede bone development, it is liable to contribute heavily to psychomotor uncoordination. This is the reason I'm not keen on preteens being on active and vigorous weight-training programs.

Even in rapid growth, the process is very delicate and precise. The body is special in the way it is able to adapt to this process. This is called normal.

The vast majority of children I see complaining of growing pains are in their very active formative years, mostly between six and fifteen years old. The sudden jars, bumps and lumps of vigorous play often produce stress on the spine, and cause the vertebrae to become subluxated. These subluxations affect the way certain nerves control the function of your child's legs, knees, feet, etc. In adults this is called sciatica – pain in the legs. Even the internal organs can be affected, creating a plethora of difficulties ranging from abdominal cramps, diarrhea and/or constipation, etc.

As well as vertebral subluxation, children can also suffer from what I refer to as a "functional pelvic imbalance." In simple terms, it is a functional error in the manner with which the pelvic bones move and function, which then changes the way a child walks, moves, etc. This subluxation pattern seems to be prevalent in five to fifteen-years-olds and can cause considerable strain on some of the muscles and ligaments of their legs. They become slightly inflamed and produce discomfort. The discomfort your child experiences in the legs, is either from sciatic nerve involvement or from continuous strain on the muscles and ligaments – *not* from growing.

These pelvic imbalance errors often cause children to develop scoliosis (spinal curvature) and change the function of certain pelvic muscles to produce internal rotation of the leg, such as commonly called "pigeon toes," or "fallen arches." To that end, many specialists have recommended arch supports, orthotics, etc. As a result, because the actual problem is not addressed, these appliances produce strain on the hip, knee, and ankle joints. This can sow the seeds of early arthritic degeneration. Not a god thing! These are often the children who are labeled as "klutzy."

Many parents are surprised to learn that most of the problems I see in adults can be traced to some childhood injury or incident, which caused a vertebra or pelvis area to become subluxated. I have just completed a seven-year research study on these phenomena. My team and I have found a new subluxation affecting the manner in which the pelvic bones function. We refer to this as a "Pelvic Distortion Subluxation." We have found it to be a major contributor to the production of scoliosis in children, leg pains, ankle inversion, feet turning in, knee problems, and a variety of other complaints children are often plagued with.

Consider this – those of you who are bothered by low back pain and leg pain as adults most likely also experienced "growing pains" when you were young. You may not have realized that by having your subluxations corrected as a child may very well have eliminated what you are experiencing today. If your child is experiencing pains in the legs, or "restless" legs, or any of the problems I have mentioned above, a visit to your family chiropractor should be a top priority.

As well as seeing a chiropractor, which I consider to be most important, the following will also offer temporary relief in the meantime.

1. Hot damp compresses on the outer part of the thighs.
2. Gentle leg stretches (your chiropractor will advise you on this).
3. Vitamin B complex.
4. Calcium supplementation.

One thing you should keep in mind is that pain is a warning. It is the body's way of letting us know that something is not right. If your child is complaining, please remember that there is a reason for it. Make sure that your children are checked by a chiropractor without delay.

18. Digestive Health

Crohn's Disease, Ulcerative Colitis, and Irritable Bowel Syndrome

I simply cannot believe the numbers of people I see at our Centre with digestive problems. Most of these patients feel that their difficulties are just an inconvenience. That they can get by with only the occasional stomach cramping, the occasional constipation, and the weekly-only diarrhea! Many hold the belief that rectal bleeding is normal, that blood in the stool is OK, and that missing school and/or work because of these difficulties is just part of life. I hate to burst your bubble, but I would like to be emphatic here. *It's NOT!*

Many people don't really understand that symptoms of digestive distress usually are indicators that there is a malfunction within the system somewhere. Ignoring such signs is akin to cerebral constipation. Such thinking doesn't handle the reason for these symptoms. One thing I have learned over the last 30 years of practice, from being involved in research, and from teaching, is that the body does not like to be ignored (Please refer to Chapter 3 for a more in-depth explanation of what symptoms mean.)

Let's take a look at your digestive tribulations more closely.

Believe it or not, your digestive system is essentially a long tube that starts at your mouth and ends at your other end. It has one purpose—to extract nutrients and energy from the foods we eat. Your digestive organs: esophagus, stomach, liver, gall bladder, intestines, etc., are simply modifications of that tube. Certain digestive enzymes, juices, acids, and other additives are secreted into this system to make the digestion of foods, and thus, the extraction of energy more productive.

This system is very efficient as long as it is functioning normally. Many children and adults, however, suffer from a malfunction of their digestive system. In fact, the three most common conditions affecting intestinal function that I saw in my practice were: ***Irritable Bowel Syndrome(IBS), Ulcerative Colitis,*** and ***Crohn's Disease.*** Although not exactly the same, they all have a great deal in common and escalate in severity.

Crohn's Disease, the most serious, is a very chronic and long-term ulceration of the digestive tract. It usually extends though the wall of the intestine and involves all layers of your "digestive tube." In essence, the system attempts to heal the localized ulcers and sores, and tends to produce scar tissue. As an end result, this can literally restrict the movement of food through the system. These are referred to as strictures. On the other hand, Ulcerative Colitis mainly involves only the internal layers, called the "mucosa," and the "submucosa." IBS is even lesser on this scale.

Patients affected by these conditions can suffer chronic diarrhea, rectal bleeding, abdominal cramping, severe pain, fever, fatigue, loss of appetite, loss of weight, malabsorption, malnutrition, headaches, etc. It has been noted that Crohn's Disease and Ulcerative Colitis increase the risk of colon cancer by as much as twenty times. This can also be said for IBS to a certain degree. If left untreated, bowel function slowly deteriorates and can be life threatening. Definitely conditions that should be avoided at all cost!

The most common medical treatment for these conditions is anti-inflammatory and antispasmodic medication, surgery, diet, counseling, etc. While sometimes necessary, this type of approach does not really deal with the *cause* of these problems, instead it addresses mostly just the symptoms. As a chiropractor, I see these conditions in a different light. One needs to remember that we are dealing with human beings, not simply their intestines. Our approach recognizes that difference.

Many people, for instance, are surprised to learn that the body is a self-healing and a self-regulating organism. In other words, it is designed to heal itself and regulate its own functions. (I covered this fact earlier in the book.) You probably have not given this much thought, but you are on "auto-pilot." For example, the cells in your digestive tract deteriorate continuously and are replaced by brand new cells doing the same function. This is normal and is controlled by your internal "auto-pilot," your own nervous system. In the case of Crohn's Disease, for example, cells in the intestine die, but are not necessarily replaced by new healthy cells. This is why the intestine eventually deteriorates and ulcerates. This can be life threatening.

One must also remember that your nervous system runs your whole body and all of its functions: your immune system, your heart, your healing ability, etc., including your digestive system. All these function under direct orders from your nervous system. It therefore stands to reason that if there is an interference with the normal function of your nervous system, your body will not work the way it should – it will start to do its own "thing." A number of studies have actually shown that this is exactly the case with Crohn's, Ulcerative Colitis, and IBS; that these conditions are neurologically based. This means that the nervous system is no longer able to control the normal function of your intestinal area.

As a chiropractor, I am mainly concerned with reestablishing the normal function of the nervous system so that the body is able to heal itself. It's that simple. For those reading this book, you may be surprised to learn that a subluxation, which has caused this scope of damage, has become a pattern in the body, a habit – and a bad one! A chiropractor who attempts to deal with this habit will, in all likelihood, place a patient suffering with these conditions on a very intense schedule to start with. The reason is to be able to change this habit. The goal here is to correct the subluxation and care should be directed at correction, *not simply feeling better*.

My experience has shown that it can take anywhere from six months to three years for correction of a subluxation that has produced this scope of damage. Therefore, it is important to be patient. The results will speak for themselves. People affected by these conditions have responded very well with chiropractic care. I am including a few letters from my patients who have gone through our Centre's program and have recovered, so that their words may add a touch of reality to what you are reading.

As well as seeing a chiropractor, which I feel is crucial, there are a number of things you can do for your child or yourself on your own:

- A *hot water bottle* placed on the stomach area will relieve much of the abdominal cramping your child may be experiencing.

- *Charcoal tablets* will help absorb excess gas if your child is bloated. Do not use for a prolonged time though, as they also absorb most of the nutrients from the digestive tract.

- *Slippery elm* will often relax the intestinal muscles and reduce cramping.

- *Multi-vitamin and Mineral complex* that contains copper, manganese selenium and potassium is very important because Crohn's, etc., are characterized by malabsorption. (I recommend "Complete" distributed by Awareness Corp. that includes 180 vitamins and nutrients.)

- *Vitamins E* is essential in the repair of epithelial tissue of the intestinal tract and acts as an antioxidant.

- *Vitamin A,* at approximately 50,000 IU per day unless you are pregnant, may be taken in capsule form, but I suggest raw carrots that have been put through a juicer. The carrots should be peeled as the skin contains most of the chemicals and pesticides that can irritate your intestine.

- *Calcium and Magnesium,* at least 2,000 mg daily.

- *Vitamin C,* in very high doses combined with bioflavonoids is essential as it minimizes inflammation.

- *Garlic,* is known for preventing free radicals from attacking the intestinal lining.

- *Vitamin B12 and Folic acid.*

- *N-acetylglucosamine (NAG),* protects the intestinal lining from enzymes that could damage it.

- *Drinking lots of fluids,* herbal teas, cabbage juice, eating papaya seeds, while avoiding stress, chocolate, alcohol, carbonated drinks, are all essential.

The above will help you and your child deal with these conditions a little easier, but the number one recommendation I could make is to see your family chiropractor without delay!

***

Dear Dr. Ressel,

I would like to take this opportunity to express our deep gratitude to you and your staff for helping Andrew and me. Although you treat our entire family it is because of our efforts to help Andrew that we are now your regular patients. Andrew, now 19 years old, had been suffering with a severe case of Crohn's Disease for most of his young life. Andrew was only diagnosed at age 14, after a doctor improperly prescribed laxatives, which caused Andrew to get severely worse.

Andrew needed four serious surgeries to remove life-threatening blockages in his small bowel caused by repeated scarring from Crohn's disease attacks. I also have been diagnosed with Crohn's disease ocalized, so far, in my Duodenum. I was diagnosed five years ago at the age of 40. I learned of your Wellness Centre from a good friend at work who also suffered from the same kind of Crohn's as Andrew but had been helped by you. Of course we were intrigued about a "cure" but very skeptical. We decided to investigate.

Before I would send my son to visit Dr. Ressel, I first visited to check out the practice and staff myself. My first visit to see you was extremely positive and professional. You agreed that we could outline a pragmatic (step by step) plan for Andrew and me to allow our bodies to heal ourselves and judge the results.

Well, Doctor, it has now been a year since we first started visiting your clinic and I think it is a fair point in time to tell you that both Andrew and I are no longer suffering from any effects of our Crohn's disease. I cannot tell you how happy it makes us to see Andrew actually leaves the house after ten years plus of suffering, to have a life of pain free fun with his friends. In my case I can now enjoy a "normal" life which one cannot appreciate until only after you lose it.

Although in Andrew's and my case, we have not conducted a scientific double blind research project ruling out all the other potential factors, we sincerely believe that your treatment is a major significant cause of our recovery and we cannot thank you enough.

-Chris Beaver

I am writing this letter to explain the conditions that first brought me to see Dr. Ressel, and the changes in my personal health situation since. I was first diagnosed with Crohn's disease when I was 19 years old. I was treated as they normally treat patients with this stomach disorder through the use of steroid medication. While this medication in the short term had some positive effects on my situation, the long-term effects were severe. Side effects from the medication included joint deterioration, as well as an assortment of long-term infections from prolonged use. The long-term treatment with this type of drug was proving to be harmful, almost as bad as the effects of the disease itself. Consequently, over the last six years, other than the typical symptoms from Crohn's, I underwent six operations for Crohn's disease and also from the side effects of the medicine; the longest hospital stay lasting 39 days!

Ten months ago I heard about Dr. Ressel's unique outlook on the treatment of Crohn's disease. Since undergoing treatment though Chiropractic care I have experienced the healthiest and operation free ten months of my life in the past six years. I would strongly recommend Chiropractic care to anyone suffering from Crohn's disease. It has allowed me to start living a normal life again pain free. He has also given my family peace of mind, as they no longer have to worry when my next attack will be. Once again I would strongly recommend Chiropractic to anyone suffering from Crohn's disease as an alternative to conventional medicine.

-Jason Hayes

When I met Dr. Ogi Ressel, he made me laugh and Mom and had a giggle over his crazy running shoes he wore that day. I felt at ease and I thought that maybe, just maybe, I wouldn't have to suffer the pain and embarrassment my IBS was causing me.

Ever since I can remember, I would have painful episodes, mostly in the middle of the night where I would cry out for my Mom to come and help me. Of course she couldn't do much for me but sit on the bathroom floor near me and just be there. The doctors said to eat more fibre and watch my diet and I should grow out of this condition. However, I didn't and the next step would be more tests, more poking and prodding and of course, drugs.

My mom wanted an alternative to putting me through that, so when Dr. Ressel's office advertised a special seminar on Crohn's disease, Colitis and IBS, my mom attended and met Dr. Ressel. That was in June of 1999, and now 11 months later I'm feeling really good. My mom is very pleased because she says I'm eating better, so I'm not malnourished inside which in turn has caused me to grow and that has helped me to play hockey better and take a body check better. Thanks to Dr. Ressel's treatment and care, my mom is also able to have a good night's rest knowing that I'm having a good sleep too. I would strongly recommend Dr. Ogi Ressel to anyone as an alternative to conventional medicine.

-Joe Shearer

Chiropractic has helped me immensely with the effects of Crohn's Disease. Since I began chiropractic treatment, my symptoms have diminished greatly. I have been leading a MUCH more active life, spending more time with friends and doing sports. Unfortunately, by the time I started chiropractic treatment, my Crohn's Disease was so bad I had to undergo surgery, but since I had been seeing a chiropractor before I went to the hospital my stay was shorter than I thought possible! I recovered extremely quickly and was back home less than a week after entering the hospital. My life has certainly changed for the better since I began receiving chiropractic treatment. The benefits are unmistakable.

-Andrew Beaver

19. Poisoning Your Children

How many of you have felt uneasy about the quantity of diet soft drinks your children consume each day? Or special low-cal foods? Or sugar-free products? If your intuition has given you internal warnings (and moms are notorious for intuition), you are correct! As a doctor who sees mostly children, I am very concerned with the increasing use of artificial sweeteners, especially by children. The most widely used of these is Aspartame (although it is being slowly "outgrown" by Sucralose – more on that later), found in foods whose ingredients include sugar substitutes.

Aspartame was not approved until 1981, and mostly in dry foods. For over eight years the FDA refused to approve it because of the incidence of seizures and brain tumors this drug produced in lab animals. The FDA continued to refuse to approve it until President Reagan took office (a friend of Searle – the pharmaceutical) and fired the FDA Commissioner who wouldn't approve it. Dr. Arthur Hull Hayes was appointed as the new commissioner. Because there was so much opposition to this drug, a Board of Inquiry was set up. The Board essentially said: "Do not approve aspartame " Dr. Hayes OVERRULED his own Board of Inquiry.

Shortly after Commissioner Arthur Hull Hayes, Jr., approved the use of aspartame in carbonated beverages, he left for a position with Searle's Public Relations, and no one said anything!

Aspartame appears to cause slow, silent damage in those unfortunate enough to not have immediate reactions and a reason to avoid it. It may take one year, five years, or more, but it seems to cause some reversible and some irreversible changes in health over long-term use.

Methanol or wood alcohol as it is commonly called, is a deadly poison. People may recall that methanol was the poison that has caused some "skid row" alcoholics to end up blind or dead. Methanol is gradually released in the small intestine when the methyl group of the aspartame molecule encounters the enzyme "chymotrypsin."

The absorption of methanol into the body is sped up considerably when free methanol is ingested. Free methanol is created from aspartame when it is heated to above 86° F (30° C). This would occur when an aspartame-containing product is improperly stored or when it is heated (e.g., as part of a "food" product such as Jello).

Methanol breaks down into formic acid and formaldehyde in the body. Formaldehyde is a deadly neurotoxin. An EPA assessment of methanol states that methanol "is considered a cumulative poison due to the low rate of excretion once it is absorbed. In the body, methanol is oxidized to formaldehyde and formic acid; both of these metabolites are toxic." This causes what is known as metabolic acidosis. If you think that this is not a problem, think again. Body temperature hovers around 37° C, perfect conditions for Aspartame to be converted to formaldehyde. This tends to affect the retina of the eye and is not a pleasant side effect. Formaldehyde is in the same direct class as cyanide and arsenic, both deadly poisons. It is also used to embalm corpses and as a preservative in vaccines. It has no business being in your child, or you!

The recommend limit of consumption for aspartame is 7.8 mg/day (I totally don't get this - are they saying that it is OK to poison your children in small doses?).

A one-liter (approximately one quart) aspartame-sweetened beverage contains about 56 mg of methanol. Heavy users of aspartame-containing products consume as much as 250 mg of methanol daily or 32 times the EPA limit. The most well known problems from methanol poisoning are vision problems. Formaldehyde is a known carcinogen, causes retinal damage, interferes with DNA replication, and causes birth defects. Due to the lack of a couple of key enzymes, humans are many times more sensitive to the toxic effects of methanol than animals. Therefore, tests of aspartame or methanol on animals do not accurately reflect the danger for humans. As pointed out by Dr Woodrow C. Monte, Director of the Food Science and Nutrition Laboratory at Arizona State University, "There are no human or mammalian studies to evaluate the possible mutagenic, teratogenic, or carcinogenic effects of chronic administration of methyl alcohol."[52]

[52] Stream Tom, Dr. Woodrow C. Monte, www.tomstream/blogspot.com.

It has been pointed out that fruit juices and alcoholic beverages contain small amounts of methanol. It is important to remember, that the methanol in natural products never appears alone. In every case, ethanol is present, usually in much higher amounts. Ethanol is an antidote for methanol toxicity in humans.

The troops of Desert Storm were "treated" to large amounts of aspartame-sweetened beverages which had been heated to over 86° F in the Saudi Arabian sun. Many of them returned home with numerous disorders similar to what has been seen in persons who have been chemically poisoned by formaldehyde. The free methanol in the beverages may have been a contributing factor in these illnesses. Other breakdown products of aspartame such as DKP (diketopiperazine), may also have been a factor.

In a 1993 act that can only be described as "unconscionable," the FDA approved aspartame as an ingredient in numerous food items that would always be heated to above 86°degrees F (30°Degrees C). Much worse, on 27 June 1996, without public notice, the FDA removed all restrictions from aspartame allowing it to be used in everything, including all heated and baked goods. Wonderful!

Let's look at this under the microscope:

Methanol, from aspartame, is released in the small intestine when the methyl group of aspartame encounters the enzyme chymotrypsin.

Free methanol begins to form in liquid aspartame-containing products at temperatures above 86 degrees F also within the human body which is at 98.6 degrees F.

The methanol is then converted to formaldehyde. The formaldehyde converts to formic acid, an ant sting poison. In case you didn't know this: toxic formic acid is used as an activator to strip epoxy and urethane coatings. Imagine what it does to your insides!

Phenylalanine and aspartic acid, 90 percent of aspartame, are amino acids normally used in synthesis of protoplasm when supplied by the foods we eat. But when unaccompanied by other amino acids we use (there are 20), they are neurotoxic.

That is why a warning for Phenylketonurics is found on EQUAL and other aspartame products. Phenylketenurics are 2 percent of the population with extreme sensitivity to this chemical unless it's present in food. It gets you too, causing brain disorders and birth defects! Finally, the phenylalanine breaks down into diketopiperazine, a brain tumor agent.

In other words: Aspartame converts to dangerous byproducts that have no natural countermeasures. A dieter's empty stomach accelerates these conversions and amplifies the damage. Components of aspartame go straight to the brain, and cause damage that causes headaches, mental confusion, seizures and faulty balance – lab rats and other test animals died of brain tumors when tested.[53]

At a recent world and environmental conference, the Environmental Protection Agency (EPA) announced that there was an increasing epidemic of Multiple Sclerosis (MS) and Systemic Lupus caused by a then unknown toxin. It was soon discovered that the toxin in question was Aspartame. Here is how this works.

Aspartame changes the brain's chemistry and has been responsible for many neurological problems such as seizures, manic depression, rage, and violence. This methanol toxicity can mimic Multiple Sclerosis (MS) so people were being diagnosed with MS in error.

In the case of Systemic Lupus, it is becoming rampant, especially among people who consume diet soft drinks. It seems to be triggered by Aspartame, and with continued use, can be life threatening. It was found that although the disease cannot be reversed, when children get off Aspartame, those with Systemic Lupus usually become asymptomatic. Those who have been diagnosed with MS, however, when in reality the disease is methanol toxicity, have noticed most of their symptoms disappear.

If your child is suffering from fibromyalgia symptoms, spasms, shooting pains, numbness in the legs, cramps and dizziness, headaches, joint pains, depression, anxiety attacks, slurred speech, blurred vision or memory loss, they *may* be suffering from Aspartame disease and a health

---

[53] Gold Mark, Aspartame... the BAD news! MindBodyHealth 1015 S. River Rd - Unit 31 Saint George, UT 84790-2249.

professional should be contacted. The paradox is that this product is being promoted to children, especially teens, as a weight-loss sweetener. Nothing could be further from the truth. I always shake my head while watching someone finish off a plate of greasy french fries, fried fish, fried chicken, hamburger, and then drink a diet soda-pop and put an aspartame sugar substitute in their coffee to reduce calories. Nothing could be sadder. I say this because aspartame actually makes one crave carbohydrates and has been responsible for many cases of diabetes.

Dr. Roberts, a diabetic specialist and a world expert on aspartame poisoning, has stated that the average weight loss was nine kilograms in people who *stopped* taking this chemical. Dr. Richard Blaylock, a neurosurgeon, claims that it stimulates the brain causing varying degrees of brain damage. Why then has this chemical not been taken off the market? The answer is actually quite simple. Apparently the manufacturer funds the American Diabetes Association, the American Dietetic Association, The American Congress and the conference of the American College of Physicians. Need I say more?

There has been considerable public outrage over this product. So much in fact that on April 6, 2004 The National Justice League filed a number of lawsuits:

Defendants in the lawsuits include Coca-cola, PepsiCo, Bayer Corp., the Dannon Company, William Wrigley Jr. Company, Walmart, ConAgra Foods, Wyeth, Inc., The NutraSweet Company, and Altria Corp. (parent company of Kraft Foods and Philip Morris).

The lawsuits were filed in three separate California courts against twelve companies who either produce or use the artificial sweetener aspartame as a sugar substitute in their products. The suits were filed in Shasta, Sonoma and Butte County, California.

The suits allege that the food companies committed fraud and breach of warranty by marketing products to the public such as diet Coke, diet Pepsi, sugar free gum, Flintstone's vitamins, yogurt and children's aspirin with the full knowledge that aspartame, the sweetener in them, is neurotoxic. The lawsuits allege that many companies are poisoning the public.

There you have it!

For safe and sweet alternatives to Aspartame you can try fructose, herbal stevia, barley malt, brown rice syrup, honey, dark molasses, demerara sugar, and Suzanne Somers' "Somersweet." Most of these are available at your local food store. But let's get a dose of reality though; one spoon of sugar only has 16 calories. *Get real!*

While I am on the topic of poisoning your children, let's discuss an issue which is very dear to all of us. It is so dear in fact, that almost every household in the western world has it. Butter and margarine. I consider butter to be one of the healthiest whole foods you can in-clude in your diet. "What? I can hear many of you saying, Isn't butter bad for you? I thought margarine and spreads were better because they're low in saturated fat and cholesterol?

Be not deceived folks! Butter is truly better than margarine or other vegetable spreads. Despite unjustified warnings about saturated fat from well-meaning, but misinformed nutritionists, the list of butters benefits is impressive indeed.

Let's look at some of these:

- **Vitamins:** Butter is a rich source of easily absorbed vitamin A (used by the thyroid gland), needed for a wide range of functions in the body, from maintaining good vision, to keeping the endocrine system in top shape. Butter also contains all other fat-soluble vitamins (E, K, and D).

- **Minerals:** Butter is rich in trace minerals, especially selenium, a powerful antioxidant. Ounce for ounce, butter has more selenium per gram than either whole wheat or garlic. Butter also supplies iodine, needed by the thyroid gland (as well as vitamin A, also needed by the thyroid gland).

- **Fatty Acids:** Butter has appreciable amounts of butyric acid, used by the colon as an energy source. This fatty acid is also a known anti-carcinogen. Lauric acid, a medium chain fatty acid, is a potent antimicrobial and antifungal substance. Butter also contains conjugated linoleic acid (CLA) which gives excellent protection against cancer. Range-fed cows produce especially high levels of CLA as opposed to Astall-fed cattle. It pays; then, to get your butter from a cow that has been fed properly. Butter also has small, but equal amounts of omega 3 and 6 fatty acids, the so-called essential fatty acids.

- **Glycospingolipids:** These are a special category of fatty acids that protect against gastrointestinal infections, especially in the very young and the elderly. Children, therefore, should not drink skim of low fat milk. Those that do, have higher rates of diarrhoea than those that drink whole milk.

- **Cholesterol:** Despite all of the misinformation you may have heard, cholesterol is needed to maintain intestinal health, but is also needed for brain and nervous system development in the young. Again, this emphasizes the need for cholesterol-rich foods for children. Human breast milk is extremely high in saturated fat and cholesterol.

In direct opposition to all of these healthful qualities, stands margarine and assorted vegetable oil spreads. While these may be cheaper, you'd never eat them again if you knew how they were made. So ... let me tell you:

All margarines are made from assorted vegetable oils that have been heated to extremely high temperatures. This ensures that the oils will become rancid. A nickel catalyst is then added, along with hydrogen atoms, to solidify this goo. Nickel is a toxic heavy metal and certain amounts of it always remain in the finished product. Finally, deodorants and colorants are added to remove margarine's horrible smell (from the rancid oils) and its unappetizing grey color.[54] And if that is not enough, in the solidification process, harmful trans-fatty acids are created which are not only carcinogenic and mutagenic, but also difficult for the human digestive system to assimilate.

Yes, trans-fats.

Here's my favorite reason; margarine, in its processed form, is only one hydrogen molecule away from being a plastic. Would you like to spread a bit of Tupperware on your toast? No? *What a surprise!*

If you are still not convinced, try this simple experiment: Place an open container of margarine in the corner of your garage. You'll notice that it will not change over time or temperature. Flies will not attack it (they know better) and bacteria will not grow on it. Why? It is not a food.

So, here is the real question? What would you rather have: a real food with an abundance of healthful qualities or a stick of carcinogenic, bleached, and deodorized slop?

Some of you might be watching your weight and be rather hesitant to add butter into your diet. Have no fear. About 15 percent of the fatty acids in butter are of the short and medium chain variety, which are NOT stored as fat in the body, but are used by the vital organs for energy.

When looking for good quality butter, raw and cultured is best. This might be hard to find, however. Organic butter is your next best thing, with store-bought butter being at the bottom of the list. Remember what I've said about commercially-raised cows; it's worth a few extra cents to get high quality butter for you and your family.

And while I'm on this rampage, let me address another extremely common and house-hold product: Caffeine – a dangerous drug.

It is the most commonly used drug in North America. 80 percent of North Americans consume it daily. Coffee drinkers usually start out with one or two cups a day, but over time it isn't unusual for the habit to increase to between five and 10 or more cups daily. The morning coffee

[55] Malkmus George; Caffeine – A Dangerous Drug, Alive, Jan 2002, Vol 231.

becomes more than a ritual: it's a "caffeine fix" needed by the body to rebalance the blood that is out of balance because of the previous day's caffeine intake.

The major addictive substance in coffee is caffeine, a white crystalline alkaloid that stimulates the brain and artificially and chemically lessons fatigue.[55] Injected into human muscles, caffeine will cause paralysis, while 10 grams of caffeine accumulated suddenly in a human body would result in death. Fortunately, coffee ingested in the common manner of a single cup at a time is not fatal because the kidneys work overtime to eliminate this toxin and prevent accumulation. That is why most people need to go to the bathroom, restroom, toilet, after drinking coffee. However, continuous use of caffeine devitalizes the body to the point that the body cannot function without it. The adrenal glands become so over-stimulated that it takes a high level of caffeine just to feel normal. Thus a vicious cycle is created. The very thing that creates the problem becomes the "cure" and perpetuates the problem.

While not causing paralysis or death, small doses of caffeine do cause bad things to happen to the body. For instance, caffeine causes stomach temperature to rise 10–15° F, making the stomach more acidic, and years of over-acidity can lead to stomach ulcers. Caffeine causes the heart to beat faster, the lungs to work harder and the blood vessels leading to the brain to narrow, while increasing the body's metabolic rate. Studies show that caffeine consumption is related to increased bladder and stomach cancers, elevated blood pressure, aggravated diabetes and damaged stomach lining. Reports indicate that caffeine may be linked to male infertility as well as birth defects, and can even be passed through mother's milk into the nursing child.

Kurt W. Donsbach, PhD, DSc, ND, DC, once said: "Would you agree that everything you put into your body should be for the benefit and the use of the body?"

Coffee does not fall in such a category. It has no positive function. It furnishes no vitamins, minerals, enzymes or protein in the diet, but does create many problems that cause the body to expend much energy to overcome. Coffee, tea, cola drinks and chocolate all contain caffeine.

---

[54] Byrnes Stephen, Why Butter is Better. Health and Beyond Online, Earl, NC, 28038-0755.

Here is a partial list of some commonly consumed foods and products that contain caffeine. The amount of caffeine is listed in milligrams (mg) per seven-ounce cup of coffee or 12-ounce can of soda:

Products	Caffeine (mg)
drip coffee	115-117
brewed coffee	80-135
instant coffee	65-100
decaf coffee	2-4
tea, iced	70
Mountain dew	55
Coca-Cola	45
Dr Pepper	39
Pepsi cola	37
chocolate bar	30
stay-awake pill	100
cold tablet	30-200
diet pills	100
Excedrin	65
Midol	32

There are many herbal teas and coffee substitutes that can be con-sumed to benefit your body. The elimination of caffeine-containing substances from your diet can be one of the most important health decisions you ever make.

Listen – be good to your body. It is the only one you'll get!

20. Becoming Sweeter

OK … you have had it with aspartame – it's off your ingestion list. Now what? Well, there is a proliferation of other sweeteners out there that are proving to be just as bad, it appears. You have to admit – the health craze is getting to you. You are beginning to study the ingredients on products you buy (this is a good thing), you watch your figure (shape, contour, physique) in the mirror, you step on the scales, eat healthier, exercise more, etc.

Why? Because you have bought into the idea that all these things will provide you with a longer life and a better quality of that life … and you are right.

So you cut down on sweets, fats, carbs, etc., in your quest.

But, passing by the sweets section of the grocery story, you happen to pick up a nutrition bar with only 2 grams of carbs! Only 2! You are hysterical! Only 2! And it's Chocolate to top it all off! Yes! You are reduced to a babbling individual on your knees in the grocery store isle with your eyes full of rain.

You munch it down thinking that it tastes "not too bad!" You peek at the ingredients and read that it is sweetened with sucralose – whatever! Sounds close to Sucrose – regular sugar, so it must be OK. Right? Not!

Dr. Joseph Mercola wrote a wonderful article on sucralose – and many of you may not realize that sucralose is marketed as "Splenda."[56]

So … is Splenda really as safe as they claim it to be?

Listen to this: as of 2005, only six human trials have been conducted on Splenda (sucralose). Of these six trials, only two of the trials were completed and published *before* the FDA approved sucralose for human consumption. The two published trials had a grand total of 36 total human subjects. (I feel better already.) Only 36! It sure doesn't sound like many, but wait, it gets worse, only 23 total were actually given sucralose for testing and here is the real killer: the longest trial at this

---

[56] Mercola, Joseph, Secret Dangers of Splenda, www.mercola.com, July 13, 2005.

time had lasted only four days and looked at sucralose in relation to tooth decay, *not* human tolerance and human health effects.

Splenda, best known for its marketing logo, "made from sugar so it tastes like sugar," has taken the sweetener industry by storm. Splenda has become the nation's number one selling artificial sweetener in a very short period of time.

Between 2000 and 2004, the percentage of U.S. households using Splenda products jumped from 3 to 20 percent. In a one year period, Splenda sales topped $177 million compared with $62 million spent on aspartame-based Equal and $52 million on saccharin-based Sweet 'N Low.

McNeil Nutritionals, in their marketing pitch for Splenda emphasizes that Splenda has endured some of the most rigorous testing to date for any food additive. Enough so to convince the average consumer that it is in fact safe. They claim that over 100 studies have been conducted on Splenda. What they don't tell you is that most of the studies are done on animals.

There have been no long-term human toxicity studies published until *after* the FDA approved Sucralose for human consumption. Following FDA approval a human toxicity trial was conducted, but lasted only three months, hardly the length of time most Splenda users plan to consume Sucralose. No studies have ever been done on children or pregnant women. Yet parents feel comfortable having their children eat sucralose sweetened foods.

Much of the controversy surrounding Splenda does not focus just on its safety, but rather on its false advertising claims. The competition among sweeteners is anything but sweet. The sugar industry is currently suing McNeil Nutritionals for implying that Splenda is a natural form of sugar with no calories.

So, is it really Sugar? There is no question that sucralose starts off as a sugar molecule but it is what goes on in the factory that is concerning. Sucralose is a synthetic chemical that was originally cooked up in a laboratory. Let me give you the technobabble run-down: in the five step patented process of making sucralose, three chlorine molecules are added to a sucrose or sugar molecule. A sucrose molecule is a disaccharide that contains two single sugars bound together – glucose and fructose.

The chemical process to make sucralose alters the chemical composition of the sugar so much that it is somehow converted to a fructo-galactose molecule. This type of sugar molecule *does not occur in nature* and therefore your body does not possess the ability to properly metabolize it (here is where a number of people have reported bloating, upset stomach, gas, cramps after eating foods sweetened with sucralose). As a result of this "unique" biochemical make-up, McNeil Nutritionals makes it's claim that Splenda is not digested or metabolized by the body, making it have zero calories.

It is not that Splenda is naturally zero calories. If your body had the capacity to metabolize it then it would no longer has zero calories. I hope you got this fact: Your body is not able to digest Sucralose.

How much Splenda is left in your body after you eat it?

If you look at the research (which is primarily extrapolated form animal studies) you will see that in fact 15 percent of sucralose is absorbed into your digestive system and ultimately is stored in your body. To reach a number such as 15 percent means some people absorb more and some people absorb less. In one human study, one of the eight participants did not excrete any sucralose even after 3 days. Clearly his body was absorbing and metabolizing this chemical. That is what our bodies are supposed to do.

The bottom line is that we all have our own unique biochemical make-up. Some of you will absorb and metabolize more than others. If you are healthy and your digestive system works well, you may be at higher risk for breaking down this product in your stomach and intestines. Please understand that it is impossible for the manufacturers of Splenda to make any guarantees based on their limited animal data.

If you feel that Splenda affects you adversely, it is valid. Don't let someone convince you that it is all in your head. You know your body better than anyone else.

The entire issue of long-term safety has never been established. Let's look at the facts again:

- There have only been six human trials to date
- The longest trial lasted three months
- At LEAST 15 percent of Splenda is not excreted from your body in a timely manner

Considering that Splenda bears more chemical similarity to DDT (Dichloro-diphenyl-trichloroethane) than it does to sugar, are you willing to bet your health and the health of your children on this data? Remember that fat soluble substances, such as DDT, can remain in your body fat reserves for decades. And what new diseases will this cause? You'll just have to wait and see.

OK, you are thinking; "so what can I use as a sweetner that is safe?"

Many people have tried the Suzanne Somers' sweetner she calls "Somersweet." It is said to be five times sweeter than regular sugar (although a number of people dispute that fact), and minimizes the insulin-carb effect on the body. Somersweet is made of some Ogliofructose, fiber (inulin), mung bean extract (a maltose-type "sugar" produced when the beans sprout, so this is a little questionable), fructose, and Ace-K (Acesulfame potassium.)[57] That last ingredient is under careful study.

Fructose is also a good substitute for sucrose – it is made from fruit (hence the name) and does not elicit the same insulin demand on the body as does real sugar. This is sweetener that I use. Some have said that is tends to elevate cholesterol and/or triglycerides in the bloodstream although I am not aware of any conclusive evidence to substantiate that thought.

And while I am on the topic of sweets, let's touch on something that many parents give their children – because they think it is good for them. So, let's talk about fruit juice.

I suspected that drinking lots of apple juice, for example, wasn't good for children because they often filled up on juice, and they wouldn't

---

[57] *The Low Carb Luxury Newsletter*, Vol 3, Issue 2, January 15, 2002.

be hungry for meals, thereby missing vital food substances (proteins, fats, vitamins, minerals, etc). What many parents don't realize is that drinking juice is like drinking concentrated sugar and can potentially deplete the body of valuable vitamins and minerals in a manner similar to eating lots of candy or drinking lots of soda.[58]

For example, when a child eats an orange, it does so slowly, and the minerals and vitamins within the orange itself help it process the sugar. The body requires B vitamins (thiamine, folic acid, B12) and trace elements like zinc, chromium, and magnesium as well as several enzymes to process and store the sugar we eat. When a child consumes a large glass of orange juice, or apple juice, it is similar to eating five or six oranges in 30 seconds, and because most juices are pasteurized, most vitamins and other nutrients are inactivated by the high temperatures of the pasteurization process. In addition, the large amount of sugar presented quickly to the body causes too much insulin to be released from the pancreas. This over-release of insulin causes the blood sugar level to drop. The brain, now faced with an unstable supply of sugar, preferentially closes down the higher learning centers (memory, thoughts, social behaviour, etc.), and instead stimulates the more primitive emotional and motor centers of the brain to deal with this perceived "crisis" (resulting in an over-active child that is emotionally "out of control").

The child and even the adult's body responds to the stress of low blood sugar by activating the "fight or flight" sympathetic nervous system: a response that creates jerky, impulsive body movements In addition, the adrenal system is also activated and releases stress steroids in response to low blood sugar. These steroids weaken our immune system (an important reason to not consume sugar when one is fighting something) and intensify feelings of irritability, anger, and even rage (i.e. temper tantrums).

An adult's digestive and nervous system are more finely tuned and developed. The adult may notice an increase in heart rate and feel a little light headed or sweaty from consuming too much sugar, but usually the adult's blood sugar can stabilize after and hour or so. For the child,

---

[58] Johnson Susan, "Fruit Juice," *Halton Waldorf School Newsletter*, May 25, 2005.

it may take four or more hours to stabilize the blood sugar after a bolus of fruit juice, soda, or candy. Each child is different, but diets high in sugar are believed to disrupt the child's neurological development by affecting the release of neuro-horomones. Some researchers also feel that the chronic overstimulation of the pancreas by a diet high in sugar may be contributing to the increase in Type II Insulin-dependent Diabetes now seen in children.

Interestingly, the most recent newsletter from the American Academy of Pediatrics recommended that children should not drink more than 4–6 ounces of juice a day if they need to drink the stuff at all. Can't beat pure water for thirsty children!

These are the facts on becoming a sweeter person.

21. Readin', Ritin', and Ritalin
The Ritalin and Prozac Controversy

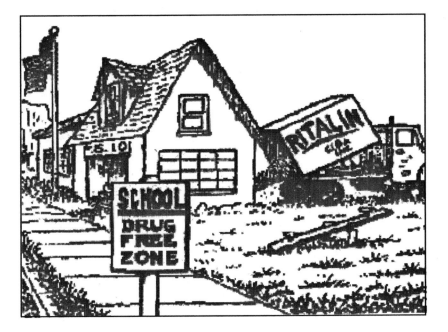

It has been called by many "Teacher's Little Helper." I'm referring to the popular drug Ritalin, which is widely prescribed to "treat" the condition A.D.H.D. (Attention Deficit Hyperactivity Disorder), commonly referred to as simply "hyperactivity."

The number of children taking this drug has risen by drastically in the last ten years or so, much to the delight of the shareholders of Ciba-Geigy (now Novartis), the drug's manufacturer. As many as 100 percent of all children (if you can believe it), in second through fifth grade, have been prescribed the drug Ritalin, even though many of them probably don't have Attention Deficit Hyperactivity Disorder. That was the conclusion of Dr. LeFever and researchers who published their findings in the *American Journal of Public Health.*[59] The United States and Canada are leading the parade in Ritalin use, while European countries are far down the list. As a matter of fact, Health Canada has recently launched an investigation to delve into the over prescribing patterns of this narcotic. Maybe children across the ocean are different? Perhaps our kids are "sicker?" Could it be marketing?

Please read on . . .

According to Dr. LeFever, doctors are overprescribing Ritalin, which is a psychotrophic drug and a Class II narcotic. "It's hard to believe this many children actually have the specific brain-related problem called A.D.H.D.," stated Dr. LeFever, an assistant professor of Pediatrics and Psychiatry at the Centre for Pediatric Research.

Health care advocates say that doctors are routinely diagnosing children with A.D.H.D., even though there are no clinical tests for this condition. Instead, they find it easier to write a prescription for Ritalin than discuss diet or parenting skills with the child's family. I really want you to get this. *There are no tests for this condition.* The diagnosis of A.D.H.D. is purely made on observation and someone's personal view of what constitutes "normal behaviour." Taking into account that approximately 20 percent of the population have antisocial tendencies, this type of criteria used to establish a true diagnosis of A.D.H.D., then sits on very perilous ground. Would you not agree?

From my perspective as a doctor, teacher, and researcher, it seems as if almost every child today is being labeled with A.D.H.D. It appears to be a catch-all name given to kids who don't fit into some-one's definition of how a child "should" behave. The criteria used to make this diagnosis fit almost every child I have encountered in practice. It probably suits most of your friends and relatives also. So much for being clinical and objective!

According to Peter R. Breggin, M.D., director of the International Centre for the Study of Psychiatry and Psychology and faculty member

[59] LeFever, Gretchen, et al, "The Extent of Drug Therapy for Attention Deficit Hyperactivity Disorder among Children in Public School," *American Journal of Public Health*, 1999, Vol 89, No. 9.

at The Johns Hopkins University, in his book *The War Against Children of Color*, A.D.H.D. tends to be a middle class diagnosis.[60]

Let's look at the factors that would label a child as having A.D.H.D.

- Often fidgets and squirms in his/her seat.
- Has difficulty remaining seated when required.
- Is easily distracted.
- Often blurts out answers to questions before they have been completed.
- Has difficulty waiting his/her turn during games.
- Has difficulty following instructions.
- Jumps from one thing to another.
- Often talks excessively.
- Interrupts others.
- Often loses things.
- Does not seem to listen.
- Has difficulty playing quietly.

If your child displays at least six to eight of these criteria, he is a candidate for the A.D.H.D. diagnosis. (All of a sudden I'm very concerned about myself, most of my friends and colleagues!)

These criteria sound like a normal, healthy, exuberant, *bored* child. Many authorities feel that these children are actually quite gifted, bright, and are very right-brained, i.e., creative. These children function with two speeds only, hyperdrive and collapse. There is no in between. They are also highly visual and nonsequential processors. In other words, they learn by pictures in a nontraditional manner.

Many feel these children are "scanners;" they scan life and the world around them in the same manner as they would scan a computer screen. Many clinicians also feel that these children are a product of our fast-paced, overstimulated culture. To that end, I must applaud the Waldorf School and their founder, Rudolf Steiner, who frown on the use of computers in their teaching methods.

---

[60] Breggin, P., *The War Against Children of Color: Psychiatry Targets Inner-city Youth*, Login Brothers, 1998.

Still others are convinced that this supposed "hyperactivity" is the result of a lack of certain nutrients and minerals. There is also a growing suspicion that the diagnosis of A.D.H.D. was actually concocted by the drug manufacturer to increase their sales of Ritalin.[61] (What a shock! I'll allow you to draw your own conclusions at the end of this chapter.)

To make my point clearer, permit me to ask you the question, "what if Einstein and Edison were on Ritalin?" If they were born today, they would surely have been labeled with A.D.H.D.; both would have been expelled from school for disruptive behaviour. Where would we have been today without their brilliance?

Most parents do not realize that this "diagnosis" is made purely on observation and is most often initiated by a teacher who is having difficulty controlling the behaviour of a certain child. I am emphatic when I stress that this is NOT an attack on teachers, rather it is an observation; many teachers have simply been misled by drug company and government promotional campaigns for Ritalin and other stimulants. "Educate – don't medicate," should be the motto of every parent or teacher who is tempted to resort to Ritalin, Breggin urges.

It is interesting to note that some teachers have very few A.D.H.D. children in their class, while it seems that others have a whole classroom. These children need a different teaching method, and this is often difficult as in most cases, schools demand obedience and conformity. Rather than use the term A.D.H.D., Dr. Breggin, in his studies on this phenomenon, called it "DADD—Dad Attention Deficit Disorder." He feels that a lack of parental attention and lack of discipline very often leads to the diagnosis of A.D.H.D. I tend to agree.

I have had the opportunity to speak with Dr. Robert Mendelson, M.D., one of the most respected pediatricians in North America, and a self-proclaimed medical "heretic" before his untimely demise, and he told me that it could be our perception that may be at fault. "Is it the child who is hyperactive," he asked, "or is it that the average Earthling is no longer excited about life?" Interesting thought!

To treat this strange, new "affliction," children are most often placed on the drug Ritalin, categorized as a Class II narcotic. To bring

[61] Citizens Commission on Human Rights, *Protesters Claim Psychiatry Targets Children for Profit*, May 26, 2000.

this into perspective, Class I drugs are those substances for which there is no legitimate use. Substances that even a licensed physician can't prescribe, eg., Heroin, LSD, etc. Class II are those substances that are also addictive but may have some limited medical value, eg: Ritalin, Cocaine, etc. Class III and IV are substances that have the potential for abuse, such as Valium and other barbiturates.

As parents, you may not realize that Ritalin is highly addictive and that is why it is placed under the same classification as cocaine. Ritalin is a psychotropic drug; it alters behaviour and a child's perception of the world. The purpose of this drug is to force the child to obey! (It also has another, more sinister purpose, which will become all too clear as you read this chapter.) I feel it robs children of their individuality and I wonder if we are not turning our children into robots!

In his book, *Talking Back to Ritalin*,[62] Dr. Peter Breggin notes that there is evidence Ritalin can cause permanent damage to the child's brain and it's function. Dr. Breggin states, "Pediatricians, parents, and teachers are not aware of these hazards, because the ill effects of this drug have been ignored and suppressed, in order to encourage the sale of this drug."

There have been few conclusive research studies done on the long-term effects of Ritalin, however, Johnson and Stewart found that:

- 83% of children had trouble with frequent lying.
- 60% of children were still overactive and rebellious.
- 59% had contact with police.
- 52% were destructive.
- 34% threatened to kill their parents. (Definitely a no-no!)
- 15% contemplated suicide.

Definitely not popular side effects! Let's look at some of the physiological effects of Ritalin use:

1. Decreased blood flow to the brain, an effect recently also shown to be caused by cocaine. It is associated with impaired thinking ability and memory loss.

---

[62] Breggin, P., *Talking Back to Ritalin,* Ingram, 1998.

2. Disruption of growth hormone, leading to suppression of growth in the body and brain of the child.
3. Possible shrinkage (atrophy) or other permanent physical abnormalities in the brain.
4. Decreased ability to learn (which is one of the reasons for the drug in the first place).

Many parents are unaware of the health problems and risks associated with Ritalin use. These include:

Central Nervous System:
- Psychosis
- Hallucinations
- Depression, Convulsion/Seizures
- Drowsiness
- Confusion
- Insomnia
- Agitation/Irritation
- Anxiety
- Hostility
- Unhappiness
- Impaired mental ability
- Tics, jerky movements
- Compulsive behaviour
- Decreased social interest/withdrawal
- Zombie-like behaviour

Gastrointestinal:
- Eating Disorders
- Nausea/Vomiting
- Cramping
- Dry mouth
- Constipation
- Liver malfunction

Endocrine/Metabolic:
- Growth problems
- Weight loss

Withdrawal:
- Evening crash
- Depression
- Worsening of the A.D.H.D. symptoms

Other:
- Blurred vision
- Headache
- Dizziness
- Rash
- Hair loss
- Dermatitis
- Blood disorders
- Involuntary discharge of urine
- Fever
- Joint swelling
- Unusual sweating

Cardiovascular:
- Rapid heartbeat
- Palpitations
- Tachycardia
- Arrhythmia
- Heart Attacks

The cardiac side effects of long-term Ritalin use sends chills up and down my spine. There are cases where a child has suddenly collapsed from a heart attack caused by long-term Ritalin use. This was the finding of the medical examiner who investigated the sudden death of a young Michigan boy[63] ... Ritalin, over time, causes changes in the small blood vessels that supply the heart muscles with blood and oxygen.

As you may have guessed, the conclusions of the medical examiner who arrived at these findings are hotly debated by a number of

---

[63] ICA News Brief, Sept./Oct. 1989, Associated Press Newswire service.

"experts." These experts feel that Ritalin is very "safe" and that there is no need for concern because such cases are rare and statistically insignificant. They are indeed. However, anyway you slice it, and play with statistics, one truth will always predominate—it is very significant to the families who lost their children! Don't you just love politics?

"Ritalin and other stimulants are currently prescribed to millions of children in the hope of improving their supposed hyperactivity, inattention, and impulsivity," Dr. Breggin warns. He presents evidence that these drugs "work" by producing robotic or zombie-like behaviour in children. This enforced docility and obedience can produce a few weeks of subdued behaviour but has no positive effect on academic achievement and no positive long-term effects at all. Contrary to claims by drug advocates, giving Ritalin to a child does not help prevent future problems such as school failure or delinquency, he emphasizes.

Ritalin's lack of effectiveness has been proven by hundreds of studies, but has not been revealed to doctors, teachers or parents. "Parents and teachers and even doctors have been badly misled by drug company marketing practices," says Breggin. "Drug companies have targeted children as the new market" – not OK!

By now you are probably wondering how this all began. It all began with Dr. Stephen Breuning who did the initial research on Ritalin. He was found to have "knowingly, wilfully, and repeatedly engaged in misleading and deceptive practices in reporting research." According to the National Institute of Mental Health (NIMH), Breuning did not conduct his research as described in his grant application, neither did he obtain the results he claimed in his report.

He was also the first researcher to be convicted for research fraud. He was sentenced to sixty days in prison, ordered to reimburse $11,352 to the University of Pittsburgh, where he worked, and placed on five years probation. The U.S District Judge who sentenced Breuning said that he "will pay dearly for the rest of his life." I am more concerned about the millions of our children's lives his "research" has touched. How about you?

"The public might be shocked to learn that the vast majority of studies for FDA approval of psychiatric drugs such as Prozac and Ritalin show them to be of no value whatsoever. The drug company researchers are allowed to pick out two, often marginally or questionably successful studies, as *proof* that the drugs work." Those are words from Peter Breggin.

Health care advocates say that physicians are now routinely diagnosing children with A.D.H.D. They find it easier to write a prescription for Ritalin and Prozac, than discuss diet or parenting skills with the child's family. Why? The public has simply accepted this "quick fix" as the norm. This is called marketing. Only in North America!

Let's look at this closer ...

You may have guessed by now that there are billions of dollars at stake. In order to promote sales of their drug, Ritalin, Ciba/Novartis has created a parent 'support' group called C.H.A.D.D. (Children and Adults with Attention Deficit Hyperactivity Disorder). This group received funding from the drug manufacturer to increase public awareness of Ritalin as a treatment for A.D.H.D. and furthermore, to suppress any alternatives. There are approximately 700 chapters of this organization across North America. C.H.A.D.D. conducts most meetings in schools, giving them an image of legitimacy and government sanction. It does not provide parents with information about A.D.H.D., mostly about the benefits of Ritalin. As well, it does not reveal its conflict of interest ties with Ciba/Novartis. The information they disseminate has helped honest practitioners harm our children – not OK!

Wait, there is more ...

One of the functions of C.H.A.D.D. was to promote the concept that Ritalin should be available as a nonprescription drug. In other words, any one could walk into a drug store and obtain it legally. Imagine for a moment, if you will, your ten-year-old buying narcotics at the corner store. As it is, however, kids "trade" and buy Ritalin from each other on a mini "black market" which seems to exist in most high schools and even the primary grades, much to the delight of Ciba/Novartis. There is something not right here. Would you agree?

I am happy to tell you that there are others who feel as I do. In May, 2000, a lawsuit was filed in Texas against Ciba/Novartis. The lawsuit alleges that Ciba planned, conspired, and colluded to create, develop and promote the diagnosis of A.D.H.D. in an effort to market Ritalin for the sake of profit. Ciba/Novartis took steps to increase sales of Ritalin by the following procedures:

1. Actively promoting the concept that children "suffer" from a disease that requires narcotic therapy.
2. Promoting Ritalin as the drug of choice to "treat" this condition.
3. Supporting groups such as C.H.A.D.D.
4. Promoting C.H.A.D.D. financially so that it may propagate the A.D.H.D. fraud.
5. Distributing misleading promotional literature to increase Ritalin sales.

One other tidbit I would like to mention is that young people who tried to join the military, were denied if they had any history of Ritalin use. This is because Ritalin is a Class II controlled substance and its use is not approved of by the military. A protest march organised recently by the Citizens Commission on Human Rights, and led by Dr. Julian Whitaker M.D., an alternative medicine guru, and Dr. Fred Baughman, a pediatric neurologist, officially announced that A.D.H.D. is a "mental disorder" propagated at the expense of school children by the drug manufacturer. Dr. Baughman stated, "Twenty-five years of research has failed to validate A.D.H.D. as a disease, or as anything wrong with the child. A.D.H.D. has no biologic or scientific validity whatsoever. It is a total fraud."

So there you have it. And just when you thought it was safe to go in the water.

I thought I would take a minute here and discuss my other pet peeve — Prozac. As in the case of Ritalin, other companies jumped on the mental bandwagon in the hope of catching the proverbial buck. This latest "cure" of depression was the result of brilliant marketing efforts by Lilly Co., the drug manufacturer. Recently, however, many members of the drug cartel have stumbled onto this, as yet virgin territory that was virtually untouched. Yes, children! Prozac alters the brain's chemistry and has found its way, in increasing numbers, into the minds of our children.

You may find it interesting to learn that in a 1999 study,[64] pub-lished in the Journal of the American Medical Association (JAMA), the authors surveyed physicians who regularly prescribe to children under 18 years of age, specific serotonin re-uptake inhibitors such as Prozac, etc., even when the FDA has *not approved* them for this segment of the population. It was found that while 72 percent of physicians prescribe such drugs to children, 16 percent feel comfortable doing so and only 8 percent feel qualified. At present, approximately seven to nine million children from Kindergarten to grade twelve, are on these drugs in Canada and the United States—not OK!

Prozac, which many are familiar with, has been associated with aggressive and violent behaviour: Each one of the shootings you have read about and which occurred in high schools, have been linked to children on Prozac or other psychotropic drugs. A recent issue of *Lancet*, a major scientific research journal, found that Prozac has been associated with increased rate of seizures, convulsions, paranoid psychosis, and suicide.[65] These are not pleasant side effects!

Why is this happening?

These drugs are being disguised and cleverly marketed to parents as health care; something which will help make their children "better." Parents are told that their child has a "chemical imbalance" in

---

[64] Rushton J., "SSRI use common in children," *JAMA*, May 26, 1999, vol. 281, No. 20.

[65] Bourguignon, R., "Dangers of Fluoxetine (Prozac)," *Lancet*, January 18, 1997.

the brain and needs these "chemical balancers" to be healthy. Noted child neurologist Dr. Fred Baughman is outraged at the psychiatry profession stating that they essentially work for the pharmaceutical industry to promote legal drug trafficking. He feels that the A.D.H.D. "diagnosis," for example, is fraudulent, and only exists so that normal children can be placed on addictive psychotropic drugs for the sake of profit.

Dr. Baughman feels strongly that A.D.H.D., Conduct Disorder (C.D.), Oppositional Defiant Disorder (O.D.D.), Severe Emotional Disability (S.E.D.), Learning Disabilities (LDs), and every single psychiatric "disorder" (those they so stridently represent to us as diseases due to chemical imbalance in the brain), are not diseases at all, but inventions, contrivances, illusions of disease. They are the stuff of labeling, drugging, and billing. It is that simple, that unimaginable, that heinous."

It was Hitler who said, "if you tell a lie long enough, eventually it will be believed as truth, and the greater the lie, the more people will believe it." Remember that Holocaust victims were marched into gas chambers for reasons of "public health" and "disinfection."

Testifying before the 1998 Consensus Conference on A.D.H.D., William Carey, President of the Citizens Commission on Human Rights, stated, "A.D.H.D. appears to be a set of normal behavioural variations." Dr. Baughman on the other hand, wrote in the Journal of the American Medical Association,[66] "Once children are labeled with A.D.H.D., they are no longer treated as normal. Once a psychotropic drug courses through their brain and body, they are, for the first time, physically, neurologically, and biologically abnormal."

Wait, it gets better ...

You may not realize this, but the fourteen-year patent on Prozac is about to expire. As you may have guessed, Lilly Co. has finally agreed with the rest of the world in admitting that there are serious problems with Prozac just as competitors are on its heels to produce

---

[66] Baughman, F., "Treatment of Attention Deficit/Hyperactivity Disorder," *Journal of the American Medical Association*, April 28, 1999, ADHD Fraud website: http://home.att.net/~fred-alden.

cheaper versions of the same drug. But, lo and behold, Lilly has announced that it now has a "new, improved" version of Prozac—one with fewer side effects! Amazing!!! Lilly has apparently known for years that suicide and attempted suicide were serious complications for people taking Prozac. It was alleged that they attempted to alter records to minimize these effects. For example, attempted suicide was changed to depression.

I do not believe that mind-altering drugs are an appropriate approach to helping our children. Instead, I urge parents and teachers to learn to identify and meet the individual needs of the children in their care.

There has to be a better way!

Chiropractic doctors have been successfully helping A.D.H.D. children and patients with depression for years. You may not be aware of this but in the 1940s, 50s and 60s there were a number of Chiropractic Sanatoriums established so that people with mental difficulties could actually get well. We often find that interference to the function of the nervous system, caused by a vertebral subluxation in the spine, is at the heart of the matter. These vertebral subluxations are often the result of a difficult birth or other trauma and interfere with normal nervous system function. This error then changes perception and, as a result, behaviour.

A vertebral subluxation is an irritant to the nervous system. It is similar to having a pebble placed in your shoe that you can't get rid of! Chiropractic care is directed at correcting these subluxations thereby making the child's nervous system function normally. It's that simple. It is for this reason that it is absolutely imperative to check children for subluxations. In other cases, this behaviour could be the result of parenting, diet, heavy metal toxicity, or simply just being a kid; let's not forget that last one. If your child has been labeled with A.D.H.D. or depression, or is in the process of being labeled, my suggestion would be to consult a chiropractor without delay.

Here are some suggestions parents might find helpful.
a. Have your children checked for subluxations.
b Talk with your children; I find that open dialogue is a wonderful way of defusing a potentially explosive situation.
c. Spend time with your children.
d. Talk with your friends and support groups; you are not alone.
e. Do not allow your child to be labeled; often children and their parents tend to live up to that expectation.
f. Obtain as many opinions as needed; you'll find a wide variety.
g. Get a hair analysis performed for toxic heavy metals as these can often cause altered behaviour.
h. The following nutritional supplements are helpful. All of these have a calming effect on the nervous system.
  1. Vitamin B Complex
  2. Vitamin B3, B5, and B6
  3. Vitamin C
i. Gamma-aminobutyric Acid(GABA)
j. Valerian root extract

There have been several theories proposed to make sense of the A.D.H.D. "thing." In their national best-seller, *The A.D.D. and A.D.H.D. Diet!*, authors Rachel Bell and Dr. Howard Peiper have challenged traditional thought and suggested that children afflicted with this "condition" are deficient in many nutrients.

These authors feel that the following are essential for normal brain metabolism:

  1. Trace minerals
  2. Digestive enzymes
  3. Essential fatty acids (omega-3)

Although I feel that the majority of Earthlings would benefit from supplementation in these groups, they are especially important for children with cognitive and behavioral "difficulties."

***

Dear Dr. Ressel,

I was diagnosed as depressed by my family doctor three years ago. Initially, I resisted taking any medication but I finally had no choice but to begin. Matters became worse and last year I spent five weeks in the Joseph Brant Mental Health Centre, an experience that I would never forget. Whilst in the hospital I took numerous types and combinations of drugs and to date I have probably tried most of them.

For a time I felt better, but earlier this year all the old problems returned and I was put on the waiting list to go back into the hospital. These were truly dark days where there was no pleasure in life and I just existed from day to day. I could not sleep and was constantly tired. I could not concentrate at work and eventually left my job. I burst into tears at nothing and I avoided seeing people and even answering the phone. I was overcome with a tremendous sense of despair.

My wife encouraged me to attend a seminar held by Dr. Ressel and reluctantly I accompanied her. She urged me to make an appointment at his clinic and whilst I was very sceptical I felt that there was nothing to lose by going. I have now been attending the Centre for six weeks and what a transformation! Although I have some way to go yet, there is now a purpose to life and I look forward to a full recovery. For the first time in a long while I now sleep at night. I never did go back to the hospital.

-Malcom Moss

The past several years have been a trying experience for my husband and me. We have been trying to find help for our son, first through the public school system, where we were advised that he go through a battery of tests including psycho-educational, auditory and visual testing. This eventually led us to seek the help of a pediatric psychotherapist, who sent him for more invasive testing through an EEG and MRI. Throughout early public school, Ryan struggled to comprehend in large classes where the teachers were not only dealing with several children struggling academically but many behavioural problems as well, with no educational assistants! But, we won't go there!

By mid-grade four we could see that Ryan was falling through the cracks, and were asked to consider putting him on Ritalin so that he could cope in his surroundings. Instead of drugging our son to cope, we withdrew Ryan from Math and Language Arts classes and I taught him those subjects at home while he attended school part-time for the other subjects and for socialization. Ryan also started the Discovery Program, a one-on-one program aimed to strengthen his deficits. Two and a half years have passed; Ryan has caught up academically with his peers.

Although his academics have improved immensely with one-on-one instruction, his ability to comprehend in an even larger class-room (35 students) really concerned me. My husband read information I had copied off the Internet regarding chiropractic care, and told me that a client of his, whose daughter was experiencing the same difficulty, referred him to you some time ago. A phone call to you was all it took to make major changes in all of our lives, especially Ryan's. Since Ryan has been seeing you we have noticed a great sense of calmness within him. He is no longer agitated over little things, like having to sit in the back seat, not getting his juice first or whose turn it is to take the dog for a walk. When he is sent to his room for three things, he comes back with three things! We now have no more yelling through the house, "What was I supposed to get?' He is much more organized, helpful, caring and thoughtful. His impulsiveness has also diminished. He asks one question at a time and actually waits for an answer. His questions are making more sense and I find I am not saying to him, "Well, what do you think?"

We recently had a family reunion at our house and instead of Ryan being constantly in the forefront (being a nuisance), I found him very thoughtful and considerate. He looked out for the children's needs and wants and put his own on the back burner. This wasn't Ryan a few short weeks ago! Our guests even noticed a big change in him. Not only have you brought a greater sense of calm to Ryan and our family, you have alleviated Ryan's neck pain previously diagnosed as 'muscle spasms' and "growing pains." It has been almost one month since Ryan's first adjustment. He is much happier, content, better focused and seems to be more coordinated. He looks forward to his appointments with Dr. Ogi and so do I, as I can see for myself that we have finally found an answer to Ryan's wellbeing.

-Brenda Hunt

Since I have been coming to see you, I have felt great. If we go grocery shopping I bring the groceries in without anyone asking me to do it. I feel more helpful and I do what I am asked to do, usually the first time I am asked. My typing has improved. I can type with both hands now instead of one. I am not as hyper now. When my neighbour comes over I don't ask her a bunch of questions any more, and I wait for answers to questions I ask. I have had a lot of pain in my neck and I don't have spasms since I have been coming to you. When I play soccer, I play better now. I concentrate where the ball goes and focus better on the game. I think I am doing way better than before I came to see you. Thanks.

-Ryan Hunt

22. Cell Phones and Kids
The Controversy

I'm certain you've heard rumblings and rumours that cell phones aren't quite as safe as the manufacturers would like you to believe. If you've been feeling uneasy about your 12-year-old "tween" having her own purple cell phone, you are to be congratulated for your insight.

There are a number of studies which point to DNA and genetic cellular damage from cell phone use – specifically EMF – electromagnetic frequencies.

So let's look at some of the research on this: In 2000, the Journal of the National Cancer Institute published an article titled "Markers of DNA repair and susceptibility to cancer in humans: an epidemiologic review." The authors summarized all of the published epidemiologic studies on DNA repair in human cancers through 1998 that addressed the association of cancer susceptibility with a defect in DNA repair capacity. I know that this seems a bit tekkie but what it means is that the NCI established a link between cancer and a defect in the cell DNA repair capacity.

Dr. George Carlo in his book, *Cell Phones, Invisible Hazards in the Wireless Age, An Insider's Alarming Discoveries About Cancer and Genetic Damage* summarized the evidence that the radiation plume from cellular phones:

1. Interferes with cardiac pacemakers.
2. Breaks down the blood-brain-barrier, which allows excitotoxins and other substances to adversely affect the brain.
3. Cellular phone radiation creates cellular micronuclei, the biological marker for cancer susceptibility.

Who is he? Dr. George Carlo is a public health scientist, epidemiologist, and lawyer who was the chief research scientist investigating the safety of cellular phones for the cellular phone industry. Therefore, he was the ultimate insider into the $200 billion per year cellular phone industry.

Dr. Carlo noted the relationship between the presence of micronuclei (each cell is allowed only one nucleus – these cells are said to have many) and cancer is so strong that doctors from around the world are using tests for the presence of micronuclei to identify patients who are likely to develop cancer. All tumors and all cancers are the result of genetic damage, and most often that damage includes the formation of micronuclei.

He is most concerned about the recent trend to market cellular phones to children. He presents evidence that radiation from cellular phones penetrates younger skulls far more deeply than those of adults. The radiation penetration of the skull for ten year olds was more than half way through the brain. The radiation penetration of the skull for five year olds was nearly complete through the brain. Dr. Carlo concluded:

1. The skulls of young children are "the most vulnerable to the risks of radiation."
2. The radiation plume that emanates from a cell phone antenna penetrates much deeper into the heads of children than adults, and these children are "more susceptible to genetic damage."[67]

These findings are echoed by Dr. Alan Preece, head of biophysics at Bristol Oncology Center. He feels that mobile phones may cause damage to health by speeding up the brain's response times. Consumer concerns mount that prolonged mobile phone use could lead to problems ranging from headaches to tumors, a recent study showing an alarming rate of brain cancer in some cell phone users is helping swing scientific opinion in Britain.

Dr. Alan Preece, is among a group of scientists becoming increasingly convinced that radiation from cell phones triggers chemical processes in the body that may be harmful.

[67] George Carlo, *Cell Phones, Invisible Hazards in the Wireless Age, An Insider's Alarming Discoveries About Cancer and Genetic Damage*, Carroll & Graf, 2001.

Six separate studies now indicate that brain response times speed up when people are exposed to radio frequency (RF) signals from mobile phones. "Perhaps we now have to accept there is an effect on the brain," Preece told a London conference on the health risks of mobile phones.[68]

In view of the controversy, here is the best advice that I can give you; keep the antenna away from your body by using a phone with a headset or earpiece, and children under the age of ten should not use wireless devices of any type. Even with a headset, if you use the phone is your car, the metal cage of your car acts like a giant antenna and the EMF are reflected inside.

In his openings remarks at a conference hosted by the World Health Organization (WHO) on Tuesday, July 12, 2005, Dr. David Butler-Jones, warned that Canadians (and others) "should moderate the use of cell phones – until science overcomes nagging uncertainties about long-term health effects."[69]

The cell phone industry is targeting children – early teens – with popular images of Barbie, Disney characters and even Hilary Duff – not OK!

Why are they doing this? Take a wild guess – money. It is a megabillion industry ... And children are the market!

My suggestion is to be very cautious.

---

[68] LONDON (Reuters), "Mobile Phones May Do Harm by Speeding Up Brain," Friday, Sept 21, 2001.
[69] Butler-Jones David, Toronto Star, Tuesday, July 12, 2005, Section: A1.

23. Vaccination
For Health or Profit?

One of the most astonishing revelations parents will ever make occurs when their child is injured by a vaccine meant to *prevent* disease. No one expects it. Vaccination has become such an unquestioned rite of passage that we fail to remember that this, like any medical intervention, carries significant risks and requires our full attention, *before* providing consent.

The information parents typically receive is written by the vaccine manufacturers themselves who stand to make billions of dollars annually from vaccine sales. Parents are told that the benefits of vaccination outweigh the risks but the risks are rarely disclosed. This is hardly surprising since the risks have never been properly assessed. Only about 10 percent of adverse events are ever reported and only about 1/10th of those are investigated. Perfectly healthy children receive numerous vaccines to prevent diseases, which may not pose a significant threat during childhood, only to contract these diseases later in life when complications are more common. All too often, vaccinated children end up living with vaccine-induced paralysis, autoimmune diseases, autism, severe allergies and diabetes, to name but a few adverse events. Some simply die. At this point, many parents are left to their own resources and will not receive due help because everyone involved wants to avoid legal entanglements.

Doctors, chiropractors, and others, who do wish to go public with their knowledge of vaccine risks, are invariably ostracized and punished. I have received many calls over the years from health practitioners who can no longer live with their silence, and beg to pass information on anonymously. The patient-doctor trust has shattered under the oppressive power of the pharmaceutical industry. But this is not where the story ends. This is where the story begins.

We do have choices. Empowering ourselves with knowledge is the most important action we can take to protect the health of our children. We can *understand benefits, risks and alternatives and we* can *make good health care decisions. I urge parents everywhere to pause long enough to make an informed choice. One of the most heartbreaking, and common, things that parents recount when describing their child's vaccine injury is the guilt they feel over having ignored their instincts to wait and learn more before consenting. Follow your heart, enrich your mind, and then make your decision. Read on . . .*

-Catherine J. M. Diodati, Author, *Immunization: History, Ethics, Law and Health*

I recently lectured at a World pediatric conference in Atlanta and Toronto where the issue of vaccination was thoroughly discussed. As well, I participated in a vaccination debate on National Television and I want you to realize that vaccination is a very contentious issue. Nothing in science is seen with more religious fervor and zeal. As a chiropractor who deals mainly with children and as a father of three wonderful, unsubluxated, unvaccinated, healthy children, I have great trepidation concerning this subject.

Why I am doing this? Two reasons. First, as you know from reading this book so far, I have a special Fellowship in pediatrics, have taught at the Canadian Memorial Chiropractic College in Toronto, have been involved in research, have published research articles, lecture internationally, was a staff writer for two national magazines, and currently write for the World Chiropractic Alliance Journal. Second, and most important, are my ethics. The information released to parents by health departments throughout North America is very one sided – there is yet another side that parents do not hear about, but should, *before* they decide to vaccinate their children.

I plan to spend a little bit of time on this subject because it is one that most parents find confusing. I've met a great many parents at our Center who have heard some distant rumors and "over-the-fence" musings from their neighbors, co-workers, and people they generally meet through other social interactions, that there are problems with vaccination. Many parents, upon hearing such rumors, usually consult their family physician only to be told "you can trust me – there is nothing wrong with it – this is a good thing to do" and the general party line that has been upheld by medicine and the drug cartel for years.

Many parents reading this chapter will feel uneasy. I can't say I blame you. The information will be unsettling for most of you. However, it will also give you the data and ammunition to make effective health choices for your children. That is my purpose. I would also like you to know and understand that although many of you may find this chapter a real eye-opener, nevertheless the information presented is factual, well-researched, and true. At the end, I am going to give you a number of sources and references that may help you dig a little deeper.

Vaccination has been likened to a medical "sacrament," by the late Dr. Robert Mendelsohn. He felt that it was a "ritual" of modern medicine used to control people. I totally agree.

Vaccination: The word itself conjures happy, smiling children lining up to receive their shots to keep them *safe and healthy*. Millions of parents blindly subject their children to this ritual for it apparently bestows "protection" from "bugs" out there. More and more parents, however, along with the scientific community, are beginning to question not only the validity of this protection but also its risks. (I'll give you a few examples of this in a little bit). If you are one who subscribes to the scientific "prove-it-to-me-first," random, double-blind, scientific model, you are in for quite a shock.

The *theory* of vaccination, and it is only a theory, has never been thoroughly proven or tested. Yet, it is a theory that many people hold dear to their hearts. Most of this fervor is the direct result of massive marketing campaigns by the pharmaceutical and medical industry. Don't you just feel better hearing this again? As a matter of fact, any research being done on vaccines is funded by the drug industry and there is virtually no research done on vaccine hazards. Any studies that have been done do not extend for any longer than a two-week period. Why? There are billions of dollars at stake. What a shock!

In fact, there is no system in Canada for reporting vaccine damage, and for compensating children that have been damaged by vaccination. In the United States, any vaccine damage and adverse events (reactions to vaccines) are reported to VAERS (Vaccine Adverse Event Reporting System) which then handles such problems. Any damage in Canada is often conveniently dismissed as coincidental, and parents of vaccine-damaged children are made to feel guilty, as though it is their fault their child "reacted badly" to a vaccine and is now brain damaged. Too bad!

I think most parents in your community would find something very wrong with this approach, and I agree.

This next bit of scientific "techno-babble" may be very over simplified: Vaccination is based on essentially fooling the immune system: A weakened or killed virus is introduced into the body, in the hope that it will somehow stimulate the body to produce defense agents called antibodies, which will then be able to protect the individual when the real thing comes along. Unfortunately, vaccination is plagued with many problems; immunity is not lasting, many children have serious complications, virtually no follow through on vaccine consequences, conflicts of interests, financial gain, to name a few.

If the theory of vaccination were successful, there would be no need for "boosters." Right? Wrong. Read on...

Researchers found that the body has specific "lines of defense" for handling an invading "bug." These are your skin and mucous lining, your antibodies, and your white blood cells. All of these need to be mobilized in a very *exact* sequence in order for your defense system to be most effective. Vaccination shots, however, bypass this sequence (The body is suddenly alarmed by the presence of an injected virus when it had no inkling that there was any attack imminent) and as a result do not give lasting immunity. This is one of the reasons why "boosters" are needed.

Consider this. Alaska experienced an outbreak of measles very recently. All cases occurring at a single high school where *all* students had been vaccinated against measles. As a result, the new CDC (Center for Disease Control) policy was that from now on all students should receive *two* doses of the Measles (MMR) vaccine. Brilliant reasoning!

Many parents, as well as the scientific community, are becoming uneasy regarding vaccination. There is increase evidence that vaccination shots actually impair the function of the immune system. According to Howard Weiner, a Harvard immunologist, vaccination actually "skews" the activity of the immune system.[70] He actually feels that a child's immune system needs to be "exercised," otherwise a child may be more susceptible to serious health problems later in life. This point makes total sense; what body part doesn't become stronger if it is exercised?

The childhood diseases such as measles, mumps, chicken pox, etc. actually exercise a child's immune system. In an adult, many of these so called childhood diseases could be serious, but in a child they actually play a very important role, which is teaching a child's nervous system and immune system how to fight off an infection on its own. This is a good thing. Vaccination, on the other hand, is passive and does not exercise the immune system. This reality may leave your child susceptible to more serious complications later in life.

We are now seeing a dangerous shift in the age group coming down with measles, for instance. Children under the age of one are getting measles, which means that they did not attain proper immunity from their mothers' breast milk. Why? The answer is that those mothers did not have the antibodies for measles. The reason for that is that they did not have lasting immunity from their own measles vaccine.

This next bit of news may shock some of you.

In Britain, and some of the other European countries, people in many communities hold measles parties, and chickenpox parties. To our way of indoctrinated, and carefully taught thinking, this probably sounds bizarre, and you may feel that this goes "against your grain." You are right. It most likely does, but, read on ...

---

[70] Weiner, H., "The Dark Side of Immunizations," *Science News*, 1997.

Parents whose children have never had measles, for instance, get together and invite a child who has measles presently. The reason these measles parties are held is so that a child may actually catch measles and thereby obtain life-long immunity. Makes perfect sense. (But you see, there is no profit in natural immunity). In North America, we have been carefully taught to fear measles, for it kills millions of children, or so the measles brochures from the drug manufacturer would have you believe. Nonsense! Let me give you a dose of reality. When was the last time someone you know died from measles? See my point?

If you as a parent feel that there is something inherently wrong with injecting your child with a gene-altering substance, your gut feeling is correct. Recent research indicates that vaccination isresponsible for the increasing number of autoimmune diseases; everything from diabetes, AIDS, cancer, autism, asthma, etc.

Vaccination has been promoted as an unassailable truth and medical sacrament. Today, however, this theory, which has enjoyed blind obedience from most of the public in the past, now has to answer some very tough questions. I mentioned that vaccination is responsible for the increasing number of autoimmune disease cases.

Bart Classen, M.D., of Classen Immunotherapies, Inc. located in Maryland, is the World's foremost expert on the vaccine–diabetes connection for instance. He feels that "the risk of diabetes and autoimmune diseases is more than *double* the benefits." The study published this past year in the British Medical Journal, revealed a 147 percent increase in the rate of diabetes seen in approximately 116,000 vaccinated children.[71] In a personal communication, he added, "the whole system of vaccination is *corrupt* and nothing more than *junk science*" … and this from the man who knows!

The vaccine controversy is hittting the popular press. In 1996, ABC's *World News Tonight* aired a special report on common childhood vaccines and the relationship to diabetes. It warned parents that the risk of this disease has increased by 60 percent in the U.S. and Finland, in children under the age of five. A special report on the relationship

---

[71] Classen, B., "The public should be told that vaccines may have long-term adverse effects," *BMJ*, January 16, 1999, 318 (7177): 193.

between the MMR vaccine and a 273 percent increase in the rate of autism has also been reported and has been the object of a Congressional inquiry by Senator Burton who concluded that there is a definite link between Autism and Vaccination.

The effects of vaccination on the production of diabetes, autism, asthma, polio, AIDS, and even cancer have become a worldwide issue. In the case of polio, for instance, statistics can often be deceptive (yes, the only cases of polio seen now are those from the vaccine itself). Most parents may not realize that naturally occurring polio has not been seen on this continent for years, even decades. The only cases of polio that exist, and there are quite a few, are from the vaccine itself. The Dominion Council of Health in Canada changed the diagnostic criteria for polio some time ago. It has been renamed and is now called meningitis. Have you heard of outbreaks of meningitis lately? This is not to suggest that the polio vaccine has not had an effect on the disease, but merely to demonstrate that there may be certain lurking variables that the health department has not made you aware of when it informs parents that polio has been eradicated because of vaccination. Ah, the games we play.

Many proponents of vaccination argue that by definition vaccination aims at "providing immunity without manifesting the full disease." The answer to this statement would be that either vaccination fails to meet its own proposed aim or challenges its own definition. As an example, in 1955, the inactivated polio vaccine caused at least 260 cases of poliomyelitis in people. Most of these (192) were paralytic in nature. In other words, people were actually paralyzed from the vaccine, and there were ten deaths. Since that time, the new oral polio vaccine that has been used has been responsible for almost every case of poliomyelitis in Canada and the United States. In fact, a New York father was recently awarded a successful verdict to a twenty-year-old case where he contracted polio and was paralyzed after changing his child's diaper.

In the case of cancer, there is very disturbing research evidence indicating that polio vaccines given to over 100,000 Canadians and Americans in the early 60's contained a certain monkey virus called SV40. This virus is now being harvested from people affected with cancer. It is thought to be responsible for many forms of tumors that seem to be defying modern treatment methods. The bigger concern, however, is that this virus has been discovered in cancers of children who have not had the original polio vaccine. This means that the SV40 virus may be spreading.

Here is an article by Shelly Page from the Ottawa Citizen published on April 6 2002 which you will find interesting:

Cancer linked to vaccine fouled by monkey virus Polio inoculation

OTTAWA - An increasing number of medical researchers believe a monkey virus that contaminated polio vaccine in the 1950s and early 1960s is causing cancer among the millions of Canadians who got the vaccine.

Researchers at first thought Simian Virus 40 (SV40) was linked only to rare brain, bone and lung cancers. But last month, two studies in the British journal, *The Lancet*, found traces of the virus in the tumours of almost half of patients with non-Hodgkin's lymphoma, a relatively common cancer in Canada, with 6,200 new cases diagnosed last year. The number of cases of non-Hodgkin's lymphoma has *inexplicably* doubled over the past 30 years. Health Canada has now said it will lead a number of studies ... that will attempt to prove or disprove SV40's link to cancer.'The issue is, does it really cause cancer in humans?' said Dr. Antonio Giulivi, the department's director of Health Care Acquired Infections. 'There is still considerable debate."

Health Canada and the Canadian Bone Marrow Transplant Group will test samples developed from about 20 non-Hodgkin's lymphoma patients at Princess Margaret Hospital in Toronto. "We want to see if we can find SV40," said Dr. Giulivi.

Canadian researchers will then study the tumours of 50 non-Hodgkin's lymphoma patients being treated at the Ottawa Hospital or in Toronto to see if they have the virus in their tumours. They will also study whether chemotherapy and other treatments alter the virus, or its presence in tumours. The team will also follow other patients with other forms of cancer to see if they have traces of SV40. Patients who have never been vaccinated have also been found to have SV40 in their tumours, adding to the mystery of how the virus is transmitted. Dr. Giulivi said they will conduct tests to see if patients were infected with SV40 during bone marrow transplants.

Dr. David Malkin, a Canadian researcher, wrote a controversial editorial in last month's Lancet saying there is enough evidence to show SV40 plays a role in the development of human cancers. "I was one of the non-believers. Now I'm a believer. There is no rational way I can figure out any other explanation for my results," Dr. Malkin, an oncologist at the Hospital for Sick Children, said in an interview. He has found SV40 in the tumours taken from families who suffer from Li-Fraumeni syndrome, which causes clusters of cancers. He says proteins from SV40 turn off tumour-suppressor genes in humans, according to Dr. Malkin. "The antigen for the virus inactivates these genes, it makes them non-functional. It's doing something that is biologically very important."

Canadian children began falling ill with polio in the early 1950s. The Salk and Sabin vaccines not only brought relief to terrified parents, but effectively ended the epidemic. Between 1955 and 1961, an estimated nine million Canadians, about half the adult population and most of the children, were vaccinated, primarily with the Salk vaccine. While it is believed that SV40 poses little risk to the vast majority of those who received the vaccines, it may still be present in the bodies of millions of Canadians."[72]

---

[72] Page Shelley, "Cancer linked to vaccine fouled by monkey virus Polio inoculation," *The National Post* on-line, April 6, 2002.

You are probably thinking, "Why did they not remove this SV40 virus from the original vaccine?" The reason this virus was not removed from the polio vaccine was that it would have been too expensive to do so at that time. I will let you formulate your own conclusions.

Despite overwhelming evidence to the contrary, most parents are still led to believe that vaccination is good for you and that there are minimal risks. Although the immediate reactions to vaccinations can be life-threatening, the long-term effects relating to autoimmune diseases may not surface for months or years to come.

If you think this cannot happen to your child, then think again. According to Barbara Lo-Fisher, President of the National Vaccination Information Center in Virginia, author, and personal friend, "when it happens to your child, the risk is 100 percent."

Edda West, who heads up Canada's VRAN (Vaccine Risk Awareness Network) in British Columbia, agrees.

In a recent and controversial issue of Money Magazine,[73] journalist Andrea Rock wrote a brilliant exposé on *"The lethal dangers of the billion-dollar vaccine business."* She stated; "with government approval, drug companies can leave your child brain dead, can spread polio from you to your child, or your child to you and can even kill you." She followed the well-traveled journalistic path of "follow-the-money."

Why would Money Magazine publish such a story? Let's think about this for a moment. Many are convinced that vaccination has little to do with health care and everything to do with wealth care, and not yours or mine. Ontario's own vaccine researcher, Catherine Diodati, agrees. She recently compiled and completed a recent study on the biomedical ethics on vaccination and published a book entitled, *Immunization: History, Ethics, Law, and Health*[74] on that same subject. This is mandatory reading for anyone with a dripping syringe!

Many are convinced that the folly of vaccination is to keep the gargantuan medical machine alive into the next millennium. This is a very sinister thought. But consider this for a moment. Medicine

[73] Rock, Andres, "The Lethal Dangers of the Billion Dollar Vaccine Business," *Money Magazine*, December, 1996.

[74] Diodati, C., *Immunization: History, Ethics, Law, and Health*, Integral Aspects Inc., Windsor Ontario, September, 1999.

a very sinister thought. But consider this for a moment. Medicine deals with disease, right? I have covered this in earlier chapters. What if everyone was healthy? Horror of horrors! There are a number of researchers that are convinced that some diseases are contrived and manufactured. After all, someone has to pay the existence of hundreds of doctors, surgeries, hospitals etc. I sincerely hope it is not you or me.

If you consider this thought a little severe, think again. Dr. Michelle Brille-Edwards, a physician and former drug safety scientist for Canada's Health Protection Branch (HPB) feels that people are dying because the Health Protection Branch is like a fast-food restaurant; it serves the client, and not is the best interest of public health. She pointed out that school vaccination forms could be thinly disguised liability forms, shifting responsibility for any vaccine reactions from the Drug Company and doctor, to the parents. They contain the clause, "I *request* that the above child be immunized," instead of "my physician wants me to immunize my child." Nice touch!

In the hope of showing you that things are not always as they seem, allow me to mention the Hepatitis B vaccine. While driving past one of our schools the other day, I noticed a sign advertising "HEP B VACCINATION FOR GRADE 7." This notice caught my eye and I felt I should write a short blurb on this issue.

Hepatitis is a liver disease seen predominantly in adults and mainly among those using contaminated needles, blood products, or among sexually promiscuous individuals. It is *not* a childhood disease, it is *not* a killer and it is *not* highly contagious, as health authorities would like you to believe. As a matter of fact there are only approximately 300 cases of Hepatitis B in North America per year – very different from the numbers quoted by health departments. Does Hepatitis B constitute a huge problem then? I don't think so.

The health department and your physician requests that your baby/child receive the Hepatitis B Vaccine to protect him/her. The first inoculation of the vaccine is given to babies. Most authorities agree, however, that a child's immune system is very immature and the benefits of this vaccine are highly questionable. In fact there has been more adverse reactions to this vaccine than cases of Hepatitis. So much so, that France has discontinued its Hepatitis B vaccine program.

The Association of American Physicians and Surgeons (AAPS) is calling for an immediate moratorium on Hepatitis B vaccines, pending further research on dangerous side affects. As well, it accused school boards requiring these shots of practicing medicine without a license. *"Children younger than 14 are three times more likely to die or suffer adverse reaction after receiving Hepatitis B than catch the disease"* it stated.[75] Dr. Jane Orient, Executive Director of the Association, went on to say, "we find it shocking that government health officials cavalierly dismiss reports of serious adverse affects as coincidental and that school officials ignore them all together. It's one thing to bar a student from school if he is carrying an infectious disease posing a threat to other children. But to require a questionable medical treatment as a condition of attendance crosses the line to practising medicine."

According to a recent federal government study, serious adverse events following the vaccination (including 48 deaths) are reported three times as frequently with cases of Hepatitis B in children under the age of 14. "We suspect the adverse reactions are vastly underreported, as formal long-term studies of vaccine safety have not been completed," says Dr. Orient. In calling for the moratorium on Hepatitis B mandates, Dr. Orient warns the increasing "vaccine cocktails" administered to children may be hazardous to health.

"Mandates effectively use school children as research targets subjected to unproved medical treatment without informed consent, in violation of the Nuremberg Code. If school administrators and government bureaucrats were subject to that code, they would be prosecuted as war criminals," says Dr. Orient.

A recent study of a national vaccine policy published in the *Medical Sentinel,* the official Journal of AAPS, exposes the secret process, stacked with special interests, that decides vaccine policies of the federal government:

---

[75] Statement of the Association of American Physicians and Surgeons to US House of Representatives Subcommittee on Criminal Justice, Drug Policy, and Human Resources of the Commissions on Government Reform.

According to Roger Schlafly, Ph.D.,[76] "The Center for Disease Con-trol (CDC) appoints members of the Advisory Committee on Immunization Practices (ACIP). The members are often nominated by the drug companies and have substantial financial ties to the drug companies. Members are forbidden to publicly discuss what happened during closed portions of the meetings. The precise scientific, medical, and political basis for vaccine recommendations is never revealed. Thus the drug companies and the CDC have strong incentives to expand immunization programs."

"We suspect financial ties between the vaccine manufacturers and medical groups such as the American Medical Association (AMA) and the American Academy of Pediatrics(AAP) which endorse the vaccine," says Dr. Orient, pointing to a substantial donation to AAP from Merck & Co., the vaccine manufacturer. She continues, "And the federal government pays the state a bonus up to $100 for every "fully" vaccinated child. What is their motive – money or medicine?" The AAPS has been the voice for private physicians since 1943. It holds that the patient-doctor relationship is sacred and that parents, not the government, should make health care decisions.

There are other concerns regarding the hepatitis vaccine. A study published just recently in the Journal of Pediatrics related that the use of thimerosal, a mercury derivative that is used as a preservative agent in the Hepatitis B vaccine and others, could add to the harmful effects of the already "unpopular" vaccine. Mercury is a "neurotoxic" agent, which means that it has a toxic effect on the nervous system – not a good thing!

Do you think that giving it to infants, whose nervous system and immune system are in the developing stages, is wise? Or is there another reason that is so heinous and perverse that it defies imagination? You be the judge.

One thing I would like you to be aware of as parents is that the Hepatitis B vaccine only lasts between seven and nine years. If that is the case then, why give it to infants? Is there some kind of worry of your child becoming promiscuous by the time they are in grade five? Or is there another sinister reason?

[76] Schlafly, Roger, Ph.D., *Official Vaccine Policy Flawed*, Medical Sentinel, Vol 4.

I thought that it is very important for you to read the article just published by Robert F. Kennedy Jr. on June 16, 2005 entitled; "Deadly Immunity" to illustrate my point: When a study revealed that mercury in childhood vaccines may have caused Autism in thousands of kids, the government rushed to conceal the data – and to prevent parents from suing drug companies for their role in the epidemic.

In June, 2000, a group of top government scientists and health officials gathered for a meeting at the isolated Simpsonwood conference center in Norcross, Ga. Convened by the Centers for Disease Control and Prevention, the meeting was held at this Methodist retreat center, nestled in wooded farmland next to the Chattahoochee River, to ensure complete secrecy. The agency had issued no public announcement of the session – only private invitations to 52 attendees. There were high-level officials from the CDC and the Food and Drug Administration, the top vaccine specialist from the World Health Organization in Geneva, and representatives of every major vaccine manufacturer, including GlaxoSmithKline, Merck, Wyeth and Aventis Pasteur. All of the scientific data under discussion, CDC officials repeatedly reminded the participants, was strictly "embargoed." There would be no making photocopies of documents, no taking papers with them when they left.

The federal officials and industry representatives had assembled to discuss a disturbing new study that raised alarming questions about the safety of ... common childhood vaccines administered to infants and young children. According to a CDC epidemiologist named Tom Verstraeten, who had analyzed the agency's massive database containing the medical records of 100,000 children, a mercury-based preservative in the vaccines – thimerosal – appeared to be responsible for a dramatic increase in autism and a host of other neurological disorders among children. "I was actually stunned by what I saw," Verstraeten told those assembled at Simpsonwood, citing the staggering number of earlier studies that indicate a link between thimerosal and speech delays, attention-deficit disorder, hyperactivity and autism. Since 1991, when the CDC and the FDA had recommended that three additional vaccines laced with the preservative be given to extremely young infants – in one case, within hours of birth – the estimated number of cases of autism had increased fifteenfold, from one in every 2,500 children to one in 166 children.

Even for scientists and doctors accustomed to confronting issues of life and death, the findings were frightening. "You can play with this all you want," Dr. Bill Weil, a consultant for the American Academy of Pediatrics, told the group. The results "are statistically significant." Dr. Richard Johnston, an immunologist and pediatrician from the University of Colorado whose grandson had been born early on the morning of the meeting's first day, was even more alarmed. "My gut feeling?" he said. "Forgive this personal comment – I do not want my grandson to get a thimerosal-containing vaccine until we know better what is going on."

But instead of taking immediate steps to alert the public and rid the vaccine supply of thimerosal, the officials and executives at Simpsonwood spent most of the next two days discussing how to cover up the damaging data. According to transcripts obtained under the Freedom of Information Act, many at the meeting were concerned about how the damaging revelations about thimerosal would affect the vaccine industry's bottom line.

"We are in a bad position from the standpoint of defending any lawsuits," said Dr. Robert Brent, a pediatrician at the Alfred I. duPont Hospital for Children in Delaware. "This will be a resource to our very busy plaintiff attorneys in this country." Dr. Bob Chen, head of vaccine safety for the CDC, expressed relief that "given the sensitivity of the information, we have been able to keep it out of the hands of, let's say, less responsible hands." Dr. John Clements, vaccines advisor at the World Health Organization, declared flatly that the study "should not have been done at all" and warned that the results "will be taken by others and will be used in ways beyond the control of this group. The research results have to be *handled.*"

In fact, the government has proved to be far more adept at handling the damage than at protecting children's health. The CDC paid the Institute of Medicine to conduct a new study to whitewash the risks of thimerosal, ordering researchers to "rule out" the chemical's link to autism. It withheld Verstraeten's findings, even though they had been slated for immediate publication, and told other scientists that his original data had been "lost" and could not be replicated. And to thwart the Freedom of Information Act, it handed its giant database of vaccine records over to a private company, declaring it off-limits to researchers. By the time Verstraeten finally published his study in 2003, he had gone to work for GlaxoSmithKline and reworked his data to bury the link between thimerosal and autism.

Vaccine manufacturers had already begun to phase thimerosal out of injections given to American infants – but they continued to sell off their mercury-based supplies of vaccines until last year. The CDC and FDA gave them a hand, buying up the tainted vaccines for export to developing countries and allowing drug companies to continue using the preservative in some American vaccines – including several pediatric flu shots as well as tetanus boosters routinely given to 11-year-olds.

The drug companies are also getting help from powerful lawmakers in Washington. Senate Majority Leader Bill Frist, who has received $873,000 in contributions from the pharmaceutical industry, has been working to immunize vaccine makers from liability in 4,200 lawsuits that have been filed by the parents of injured children. On five separate occasions, Frist has tried to seal all of the government's vaccine-related documents – including the Simpsonwood transcripts – and shield Eli Lilly, the developer of thimerosal, from subpoenas. In 2002, the day after Frist quietly slipped a rider known as the "Eli Lilly Protection Act" into a homeland security bill, the company contributed $10,000 to his campaign and bought 5,000 copies of his book on bioterrorism. Congress repealed the measure in 2003 – but earlier this year, Frist slipped another provision into an anti-terrorism bill that would deny compensation to children suffering from vaccine-related brain disorders. "The lawsuits are of such magnitude that they could put vaccine producers out of business and limit our capacity to deal with a biological attack by terrorists," says Andy Olsen, a legislative assistant to Frist.

Even many conservatives are shocked by the government's effort to cover up the dangers of thimerosal. Rep. Dan Burton, a Republican from Indiana, oversaw a three-year investigation of thimerosal after his grandson was diagnosed with autism. "Thimerosal used as a preservative in vaccines is directly related to the autism epidemic," his House Government Reform Committee concluded in its final report. "This epidemic in all probability may have been prevented or curtailed had the FDA not been asleep at the switch regarding a lack of safety data regarding injected thimerosal, a known neurotoxin." The FDA and other public-health agencies failed to act, the committee added, out of "institutional malfeasance for self protection" and "misplaced protectionism of the pharmaceutical industry."

The story of how government health agencies colluded with Big Pharma to hide the risks of thimerosal from the public is a chilling case study of institutional arrogance, power and greed. I was drawn into the controversy only reluctantly. As an attorney and environmentalist who has spent years working on issues of mercury toxicity, I frequently met mothers of autistic children who were absolutely convinced that their kids had been injured by vaccines. Privately, I was skeptical. I doubted that autism could be blamed on a single source, and I certainly understood the government's need to reassure parents that vaccinations are safe; the eradication of deadly childhood diseases depends on it. I tended to agree with skeptics like Rep. Henry Waxman, a Democrat from California, who criticized his colleagues on the House Government Reform Committee for leaping to conclusions about autism and vaccinations. "Why should we scare people about immunization," Waxman pointed out at one hearing, "until we know the facts?"

It was only after reading the Simpsonwood transcripts, studying the leading scientific research and talking with many of the nation's preeminent authorities on mercury that I became convinced that the link between thimerosal and the epidemic of childhood neurological disorders is real. Five of my own children are members of the Thimerosal Generation – those born between 1989 and 2003 – who received heavy doses of mercury from vaccines. "The elementary grades are overwhelmed with children who have symptoms of neurological or immune-system damage," Patti White, a school nurse, told the House Government Reform Committee in 1999. "Vaccines are supposed to be making us healthier; however, in 25 years of nursing I have never seen so many damaged, sick kids. Something very, very wrong is happening to our children." More than 500,000 kids currently suffer from autism, and pediatricians diagnose more than 40,000 new cases every year. The disease was unknown until 1943, when it was identified and diagnosed among 11 children born in the months after thimerosal was first added to baby vaccines in 1931.

Some skeptics dispute that the rise in autism is caused by thimerosal-tainted vaccinations. They argue that the increase is a result of better diagnosis – a theory that seems questionable at best, given that most of the new cases of autism are clustered within a single generation of children. "If the epidemic is truly an artifact of poor diagnosis," scoffs Dr. Boyd Haley, one of the world's authorities on mercury toxicity, "then where are all the 20-year-old autistics?" Other researchers point out that Americans are exposed to a greater cumulative "load" of mercury than ever before, from contaminated fish to dental fillings, and suggest that thimerosal in vaccines may be only part of a much larger problem. It's a concern that certainly deserves far more attention than it has received – but it overlooks the fact that the mercury concentrations in vaccines dwarf other sources of exposure to our children.

What is most striking is the lengths to which many of the leading detectives have gone to ignore – and cover up – the evidence against thimerosal. From the very beginning, the scientific case against the mercury additive has been overwhelming. The preservative, which is used to stem fungi and bacterial growth in vaccines, contains ethylmercury, a potent neurotoxin. Truckloads of studies have shown that mercury tends to accumulate in the brains of primates and other animals after they are injected with vaccines – and that the developing brains of infants are particularly susceptible. In 1977, a Russian study found that adults exposed to much lower concentrations of ethyl mercury than those given to American children still suffered brain damage years later. Russia banned thimerosal from children's vaccines 20 years ago, and Denmark, Austria, Japan, Great Britain and all the Scandinavian countries have since followed suit.

"You couldn't even construct a study that shows thimerosal is safe," says Haley, who heads the chemistry department at the University of Kentucky. "It's just too darn toxic. If you inject thimerosal into an animal, its brain will sicken. If you apply it to living tissue, the cells die. If you put it in a petri dish, the culture dies. Knowing these things, it would be shocking if one could inject it into an infant without causing damage."

Internal documents reveal that Eli Lilly, which first developed thimerosal, knew from the start that its product could cause damage – and even death – in both animals and humans. In 1930, the company tested thimerosal by administering it to 22 patients with terminal meningitis, all of whom died within weeks of being injected – a fact Lilly didn't bother to report in its study declaring thimerosal safe. In 1935, researchers at another vaccine manufacturer, Pittman-Moore, warned Lilly that its claims about thimerosal's safety "did not check with ours." Half the dogs Pittman injected with thimerosal-based vaccines became sick, leading researchers there to declare the preservative "unsatisfactory as a serum intended for use on dogs."

In the decades that followed, the evidence against thimerosal continued to mount. During the Second World War, when the Department of Defense used the preservative in vaccines on soldiers, it required Lilly to label it "poison." In 1967, a study in Applied Microbiology found that thimerosal killed mice when added to injected vaccines. Four years later, Lilly's own studies discerned that thimerosal was "toxic to tissue cells" in concentrations as low as one part per million – 100 times weaker than the concentration in a typical vaccine. Even so, the company continued to promote thimerosal as "nontoxic" and also incorporated it into topical disinfectants. In 1977, 10 babies at a Toronto hospital died when an antiseptic preserved with thimerosal was dabbed onto their umbilical cords.

In 1982, the FDA proposed a ban on over-the-counter products that contained thimerosal, and in 1991 the agency considered banning it from animal vaccines. But tragically, that same year, the CDC recommended that infants be injected with a series of mercury-laced vaccines. Newborns would be vaccinated for hepatitis B within 24 hours of birth, and 2-month-old infants would be immunized for haemophilus influenzae B and diphtheria-tetanus-pertussis.

The drug industry knew the additional vaccines posed a danger. The same year that the CDC approved the new vaccines, Dr. Maurice Hilleman, one of the fathers of Merck's vaccine programs, warned the company that 6-month-olds who were administered the shots would suffer dangerous exposure to mercury. He recommended that thimerosal be discontinued, "especially when used on infants and children," noting that the industry knew of nontoxic alternatives. "The best way to go," he added, "is to switch to dispensing the actual vaccines without adding preservatives."

For Merck and other drug companies, however, the obstacle was money. Thimerosal enables the pharmaceutical industry to package vaccines in vials that contain multiple doses, which require additional protection because they are more easily contaminated by multiple needle entries. The larger vials cost half as much to produce as smaller, single-dose vials, making it cheaper for international agencies to distribute them to impoverished regions at risk of epidemics. Faced with this "cost consideration," Merck ignored Hilleman's warnings, and government officials continued to push more and more thimerosal-based vaccines for children. Before 1989, American preschoolers received 11 vaccinations – for polio, diphtheria-tetanus-pertussis and measles-mumps-rubella. A decade later, thanks to federal recommendations, children were receiving a total of 22 immunizations by the time they reached first grade.

As the number of vaccines increased, the rate of autism among children exploded. During the 1990s, 40 million children were injected with thimerosal-based vaccines, receiving unprecedented levels of mercury during a period critical for brain development. Despite the well-documented dangers of thimerosal, it appears that no one bothered to add up the cumulative dose of mercury that children would receive from the mandated vaccines. "What took the FDA so long to do the calculations?" Peter Patriarca, director of viral products for the agency, asked in an e-mail to the CDC in 1999. "Why didn't CDC and the advisory bodies do these calculations when they rapidly expanded the childhood immunization schedule?"

But by that time, the damage was done. Infants who received all their vaccines, plus boosters, by the age of six months were being injected with a total of 187 micrograms of ethylmercury – a level 40 percent greater than the EPA's limit for daily exposure to methylmercury, a related neurotoxin. Although the vaccine industry insists that ethylmercury poses little danger because it breaks down rapidly and is removed by the body, several studies – including one published in April by the National Institutes of Health – suggest that ethylmercury is actually *more* toxic to developing brains and stays in the brain *longer* than methylmercury. Under the expanded schedule of vaccinations, multiple shots were often administered on a single day: At two months, when the infant brain is still at a critical stage of development, children routinely received three innoculations that delivered 99 times the approved limit of mercury.

Officials responsible for childhood immunizations insist that the additional vaccines were necessary to protect infants from disease and that thimerosal is still essential in developing nations, which, they often claim, cannot afford the single-dose vials that don't require a preservative. Dr. Paul Offit, one of CDC's top vaccine advisors, told me, "I think if we really have an influenza pandemic – and certainly we will in the next 20 years, because we always do — there's no way on God's earth that we immunize 280 million people with single-dose vials. There has to be multidose vials."

But while public-health officials may have been well-intentioned, many of those on the CDC advisory committee who backed the additional vaccines had close ties to the industry. Dr. Sam Katz, the committee's chair, was a paid consultant for most of the major vaccine makers and shares a patent on a measles vaccine with Merck, which also manufactures the hepatitis B vaccine. Dr. Neal Halsey, another committee member, worked as a researcher for the vaccine companies and received honoraria from Abbott Labs for his research on the hepatitis B vaccine.

Indeed, in the tight circle of scientists who work on vaccines, such conflicts of interest are common. Rep. Burton says that the CDC "routinely allows scientists with blatant conflicts of interest to serve on intellectual advisory committees that make recommendations on new vaccines," even though they have "interests in the products and companies for which they are supposed to be providing unbiased over-sight." The House Government Reform Committee discovered that four of the eight CDC advisors who approved guidelines for a rotavirus vaccine "had financial ties to the pharmaceutical companies that were developing different versions of the vaccine."

Offit, who shares a patent on one of the vaccines, acknowledged to me that he "would make money" if his vote eventually leads to a marketable product. But he dismissed my suggestion that a scientist's direct financial stake in CDC approval might bias his judgment. "It provides no conflict for me," he insists. "I have simply been informed by the process, not corrupted by it. When I sat around that table, my sole intent was trying to make recommendations that best benefited the children in this country. It's offensive to say that physicians and public-health people are in the pocket of industry and thus are making decisions that they know are unsafe for children. It's just not the way it works."

Other vaccine scientists and regulators gave me similar assur-ances. Like Offit, they view themselves as enlightened guardians of children's health, proud of their "partnerships" with pharmaceutical companies, immune to the seductions of personal profit, besieged by irrational activists whose anti-vaccine campaigns are endangering children's health. They are often resentful of questioning. "Science," says Offit, "is best left to scientists."

Still, some government officials were alarmed by the apparent conflicts of interest. In his e-mail to CDC administrators in 1999, Paul Patriarca of the FDA blasted federal regulators for failing to adequately scrutinize the danger posed by the added baby vaccines. "I'm not sure there will be an easy way out of the potential perception that the FDA, CDC and immunization-policy bodies may have been asleep at the switch re: thimerosal until now," Patriarca wrote. The close ties between regulatory officials and the pharmaceutical industry, he added, "will also raise questions about various advisory bodies regarding aggressive recommendations for use" of thimerosal in child vaccines.

If federal regulators and government scientists failed to grasp the potential risks of thimerosal over the years, no one could claim ignorance after the secret meeting at Simpsonwood. But rather than conduct more studies to test the link to autism and other forms of brain damage, the CDC placed politics over science. The agency turned its database on childhood vaccines – which had been developed largely at taxpayer expense – over to a private agency, America's Health Insurance Plans, ensuring that it could not be used for additional research. It also instructed the Institute of Medicine, an advisory organization that is part of the National Academy of Sciences, to produce a study debunking the link between thimerosal and brain disorders. The CDC "wants us to declare, well, that these things are pretty safe," Dr. Marie McCormick, who chaired the IOM's Immunization Safety Review Committee, told her fellow researchers when they first met in January 2001. "We are not ever going to come down that [autism] is a true side effect" of thimerosal exposure. According to transcripts of the meeting, the committee's chief staffer, Kathleen Stratton, predicted that the IOM would conclude that the evidence was "inadequate to accept or reject a causal relation" between thimerosal and autism. That, she added, was the result "Walt wants" – a reference to Dr. Walter Orenstein, director of the National Immunization Program for the CDC.

For those who had devoted their lives to promoting vaccination, the revelations about thimerosal threatened to undermine everything they had worked for. "We've got a dragon by the tail here," said Dr. Michael Kaback, another committee member. "The more negative that [our] presentation is, the less likely people are to use vaccination, immunization – and we know what the results of that will be. We are kind of caught in a trap. How we work our way out of the trap, I think is the charge."

Even in public, federal officials made it clear that their primary goal in studying thimerosal was to dispel doubts about vaccines. "Four current studies are taking place to rule out the proposed link between autism and thimerosal," Dr. Gordon Douglas, then-director of strategic planning for vaccine research at the National Institutes of Health, assured a Princeton University gathering in May 2001. "In order to undo the harmful effects of research claiming to link the [measles] vaccine to an elevated risk of autism, we need to conduct and publicize additional studies to assure parents of safety." Douglas formerly served as president of vaccinations for Merck, where he ignored warnings about thimerosal's risks.

In May of last year, the Institute of Medicine issued its final report. Its conclusion: There is no proven link between autism and thimerosal in vaccines. Rather than reviewing the large body of literature describing the toxicity of thimerosal, the report relied on four disastrously flawed epidemiological studies examining European countries, where children received much smaller doses of thimerosal than American kids. It also cited a new version of the Verstraeten study, published in the journal Pediatrics, that had been reworked to reduce the link between thimerosal and autism. The new study included children too young to have been diagnosed with autism and overlooked others who showed signs of the disease. The IOM declared the case closed and – in a startling position for a scientific body – recommended that no further research be conducted.

The report may have satisfied the CDC, but it convinced no one. Rep. David Weldon, a Republican physician from Florida who serves on the House Government Reform Committee, attacked the Institute of Medicine, saying it relied on a handful of studies that were "fatally flawed" by "poor design" and failed to represent "all the available scientific and medical research." CDC officials are not interested in an honest search for the truth, Weldon told me, because "an association between vaccines and autism would force them to admit that their policies irreparably damaged thousands of children. Who would want to make that conclusion about themselves?"

Under pressure from Congress, parents and a few of its own panel members, the Institute of Medicine reluctantly convened a second panel to review the findings of the first. In February, the new panel, composed of different scientists, criticized the earlier panel for its lack of transparency and urged the CDC to make its vaccine database available to the public.

So far, though, only two scientists have managed to gain access. Dr. Mark Geier, president of the Genetics Center of America, and his son, David, spent a year battling to obtain the medical records from the CDC. Since August 2002, when members of Congress pressured the agency to turn over the data, the Geiers have completed six studies that demonstrate a powerful correlation between thimerosal and neurological damage in children. One study, which compares the cumulative dose of mercury received by children born between 1981 and 1985 with those born between 1990 and 1996, found a "very significant relationship" between autism and vaccines. Another study of educational performance found that kids who received higher doses of thimerosal in vaccines were nearly three times as likely to be diagnosed with autism and more than three times as likely to suffer from speech disorders and mental retardation. Another soon-to-be-published study shows that autism rates are in decline following the recent elimination of thimerosal from most vaccines.

As the federal government worked to prevent scientists from studying vaccines, others have stepped in to study the link to autism. In April, reporter Dan Olmsted of UPI undertook one of the more interesting studies himself. Searching for children who had not been exposed to mercury in vaccines – the kind of population that scientists typically use as a "control" in experiments – Olmsted scoured the Amish of Lancaster County, Penn., who refuse to immunize their infants. Given the national rate of autism, Olmsted calculated that there should be 130 autistics among the Amish. He found only four. One had been exposed to high levels of mercury from a power plant. The other three – including one child adopted from outside the Amish community – had received their vaccines.

At the state level, many officials have also conducted in-depth reviews of thimerosal. While the Institute of Medicine was busy whitewashing the risks, the Iowa Legislature was carefully combing through all of the available scientific and biological data. "After three years of review, I became convinced there was sufficient credible research to show a link between mercury and the increased incidences in autism," says state Sen. Ken Veenstra, a Republican who oversaw the investigation. "The fact that Iowa's 700 percent increase in autism began in the 1990s, right after more and more vaccines were added to the children's vaccine schedules, is solid evidence alone." Last year, Iowa became the first state to ban mercury in vaccines, followed by California. Similar bans are now under consideration in 32 other states.

But instead of following suit, the FDA continues to allow manufacturers to include thimerosal in scores of over-the-counter medications as well as steroids and injected collagen. Even more alarming, the government continues to ship vaccines preserved with thimerosal to developing countries – some of which are now experiencing a sudden explosion in autism rates. In China, where the disease was virtually unknown prior to the introduction of thimerosal by U.S. drug manufacturers in 1999, news reports indicate that there are now more than 1.8 million autistics. Although reliable numbers are hard to come by, autistic disorders also appear to be soaring in India, Argentina, Nicaragua and other developing countries that are now using thimerosal-laced vaccines. The World Health Organization continues to insist thimerosal is safe, but it promises to keep the possibility that it is linked to neurological disorders 'under review.'"

Mr. Kennedy said further said; "I devoted time to study this issue because I believe that this is a moral crisis that must be addressed. If, as the evidence suggests, our public-health authorities knowingly allowed the pharmaceutical industry to poison an entire generation of American children, their actions arguably constitute one of the biggest scandals in the annals of American medicine. "The CDC is guilty of incompetence and gross negligence," says Mark Blaxill, vice president of Safe Minds, a nonprofit organization concerned about the role of mercury in medicines. "The damage caused by vaccine exposure is massive. It's bigger than asbestos, bigger than tobacco, bigger than anything you've ever seen." It's hard to calculate the damage to our country – and to the international efforts to eradicate epidemic diseases – if Third World nations come to believe that America's most heralded foreign-aid initiative is poisoning their children. It's not difficult to predict how this scenario will be interpreted by America's enemies abroad. The scientists and re-searchers – many of them sincere, even idealistic – who are participating in efforts to hide the science on thimerosal claim that they are trying to advance the lofty goal of protecting children in developing nations from disease pandemics. They are badly misguided. Their failure to come clean on thimerosal will come back horribly to haunt our country and the world's poorest populations."[77] And just when you felt safe to go in the water ...

And in a recent study, Dr. Mark Geier concluded: "In light of voluminous literature supporting the biologic mechanisms for mercury-induced adverse reactions, the presence of amounts of mercury in thimerosal-containing childhood vaccines exceeding Federal Safety Guidelines for the oral ingestion of mercury, and previous epidemi-ological studies showing adverse reactions to such vaccines, a causal relationship between thimerosal-containing childhood vaccines and neurodevelopment disorders and heart disease appears to be confirmed."[78]

You should know that the Dallas based law firm of Waters & Kraus is litigating a growing number of individual cases across the coun-try involving infants that sustained serious neurological injuries from the thimerosal contained in their pediatric vaccines.

I'm certain that most of you have heard about the SARS "epidemic" (Sudden Acute Respiratory Syndrome) that almost closed the city of Toronto, two years ago. It is thought to have been cause by a coronavirus, which causes 30 percent of all colds people get. Many people feel that this was a "manufactured" disease for the purpose of revving up the vaccine machine. You can bet your boots that the government will strongly "request" yearly SARS shots – as soon as the vaccine is made.[79]

The government is under tremendous legal pressure to offer full disclosure of the benefits and the dangerous side affects before any scheduled vaccination takes place, something that has not been done. This is called *Informed Consent*. As well, the health department is not very big on informing parents that they actually have a choice to vacci-nate their children or not. This has been conveniently hidden from the public under threats of school suspension.

---

[77] Kennedy Robert, Deadly immunity, www.salon.com, June 15, 2005.
[78] Geier Mark, Childhood Vaccines Linked to Autism, Heart Disease, http://www.usnewswire.com.
[79] West Edda, Reeving up the Vaccine Machine, VRAN, April 13, 2003.

Many parents also are made to feel that a child would not be allowed in school if he/she were not vaccinated. Not true! Our local health department has omitted to tell you that you actually have a choice and that vaccination exemption forms are available at your local health office.

Here are some suggestions for you:

- Question everything.
- Ask your doctor about side affects and whether he/she is aware of the latest research on vaccines.
- Ask for proof (not a vaccine brochure from the health department or drug company).
- Do you know how to recognize a vaccine reaction?
- Ask about the vaccine lot number.
- Ask about liability. This is actually a good question, which should cut through all the bologna.
- Finally, you may want to have your doctor sign your very own *"Consent for Administration of Vaccination"* form (included in this chapter.) It shifts responsibility for any potential reactions and future complications to the person actually administering the vaccine. If your doctor or health department representative will not sign it, beware. Remember that you have choices. You should be your child's health guardian.

Here is an example of the most conniving and diabolical machination on the issue of vaccination yet:

The College of Chiropractors of Ontario (and I'll mention these people later on in the book), those people who license chiropractors to practice in the Province of Ontario, have passed a law last year, which has made it *illegal* for an Ontario Chiropractor to discuss the issue of vaccination with patients and others. None. Niet. Nic, Zilch, Nothing. What it means is that if a Chiropractic doctor is caught discussing this issue, they will be charged with Misconduct and can lose their license. Nice!

Here is the really bizarre thing. The mandate of this College is to protect the public – that is their job – supposedly. Placing a gag order on the profession so that individual doctors cannot discuss this issue with patients – even when requested – is morally, scientifically, and clinically, unthinkable. It goes against the oath we swore upon graduation.

If you, as a parent and a member of the public, feel outraged over this regulation, I urge you to write to or call the President of the College at the address below and let them know how you feel about their "protection" and their new regulation. There is nothing like public pressure to open doors:

> The College of Chiropractors of Ontario
> 130 Bloor St. West, Suite 902
> TORONTO, Ontario, Canada M5S 1N5
> Phone: 416-922-6355
> Fax: 416-925-9610
> E-mail: cco.info@cco.on.ca

***

Dear Dr. Ressel,

I remember meeting you two years ago and thinking you were nuts. Why wouldn't any responsible parent vaccinate their child? How crazy is that? Then you handed me some information about the research and risks of vaccination; I didn't want to believe it. I wanted to find out for myself what the pros and cons of vaccination were.

I asked friends and family, researched at the library, and even contacted the Health Department. On the pro side, I found that vaccines are safe (supposedly) on a schedule that gave an infant eighteen combined shots in the first year. On the con side, I found a lot of articles, books and stories to support what you had told me. It seems you were not as crazy as I had thought!

The results scared me and sometimes I couldn't finish reading stories because I would cry so hard for the people who have a reaction, and what their life is like now. How could I possibly put my child at risk? Dennis and I took 4 months to make our decision and the hardest part was taking Megan, our daughter, for her eighteen-month check up and telling the doctor that she was not getting any more shots. I was bombarded with the question, "why?" I asked for more clinical information and was given stuff that I couldn't even understand, and wondered if the doctor had even read it. The whole time in my head I was saying, "Have I done the right thing?" With all this media and public health pressure, not to mention friends and relatives that haven't read up on the subject, it's really hard to think so. One day I decided enough was enough, I needed to find people just like me who need support, reassurance, and that, yes, what we are doing is the right thing. So I started my own support group.

I've learned to question everything, and to keep my eyes open and you are the one that taught me. I can't thank you enough for having the passion to make sure everyone you meet has an informed choice not only for vaccination but also for total health care. My hat is off to you.

-Elaine Tracz

Informed Consent Form
Consent for Administration of Vaccination

Dear Responsible Physician,

You have suggested/requested that I have my child vaccinated. Before I comply with your request, I will need you to complete the following consent form.

I *(Physician's name)* _____

do hereby state that I have advised my patient _____ ,

and/or parent of my patient _____

that in my professional opinion, this patient/child should be given the vaccine,

drug, or other *(name of vaccine/drug/other)* _____ ,

manufacturers name _____ lot number _____ .

I have on this *(day)* _____ , *(month)* _____ , *(year)* _____ administered this vaccine/drug AFTER thoroughly advising the above patient/parent that there is little or no risk involved with this vaccine/ drug. I do hereby agree that should this patient at any time, suffer or develop any permanent condition deleterious or injurious to his/her health as a result of this treatment, I will be held responsible for any and all costs involved related to the care and treatment needed for this patient for the rest of his/her natural life.

Address of physician: _____

Signature of physician: _____

Signature of person administering vaccine/drug on behalf of physician:

_____

Witness _____ Date _____

24. Arthritis and Spinal Degeneration

You are probably wondering why I would discuss this issue in a book, which is primarily directed at children's health. The sad reality is that I saw a large number of children at our Centre with the beginnings of arthritis. Some of these children were very young – six, seven, and ten years old. This is actually quite a huge problem, which I have found to be downplayed by society and medicine in general when it concerns children. No one wants to talk about it!

There are many different types of arthritis. When I mention this subject, most people automatically receive a picture in their mind of their grandmother or an older adult sitting in a rocking chair with a blanket on their knees, their hands gnarled and deformed, being unable to move or walk. This is not the type of arthritis I am referring to. I am describing osteoarthritis, most often touted as a "wear-and-tear" type phenomena which for years has been associated with aging. I am going to share some statistics and data with you so that you can be the judge of how correct our thinking has been and whether it is time to slay some of our "sacred cows."

You may not realize this, but of all the illnesses that plague Mankind, this type of arthritis is the most widespread. Research indicates that it can be detected in 35 percent of the general population by the age of thirty, although my experience tells me that to be more accurate, this number should be closer to 70 percent. By the time someone is seventy years old, this condition seems to be absolutely universal. In other words, almost every seventy-year-old on the face of the planet has it. A study by Lawrence a few years ago, revealed that osteoarthritis can be noted on an x-ray in 10 percent of fifteen-year-olds (from my experience with children, and from being involved in research, that figure should be closer to 50 percent to be more accurate.)

Let me translate that statistic for you. This means that five out of every ten fifteen-year-olds has arthritis of the spine already beginning.

Did you know that? Were you aware that this condition is so prevalent? It is a condition, which is the most frequent cause of aches and pains in people and can result in the most significant time lost from work. For years, it has been regarded as a problem with no apparent solution.

Osteoarthritis has been characterized clinically by pain, deformity, limitation of movement and eventually, by disability. Any notion or thought even remotely associated with slowing it down, stopping it, or most certainly, reversing this condition, has been looked upon, until recently, as absolute "heresy." It has been universally accepted as a simple and inescapable part of aging. If you think about this from a logical perspective, however, and if that *was* the case, then why is it showing up in children who are five, six, seven or ten years old? I will answer this question a little bit later on in this chapter.

You have most likely heard that arthritis is a "wear and tear" degeneration of some of the structures of a joint and that is absolutely correct. Something you may not be aware of is that joints in your body are areas where two bones come together for the purpose of movement. The ends of these bones are lined with a very special material called cartilage, which is designed in such a way as to prevent friction. This results in movement that is very smooth, not painful, etc. As a matter of fact, the surface of the cartilage that lines your joints is so perfect, as to be *almost frictionless*. As I mentioned before, it is a self-regenerating mechanism; cartilage has the ability to regenerate. The whole joint is then bathed continuously in a special lubricating fluid called synovial fluid, which acts much like a lubricant.

Although I am speaking of the large joints of the body, such as the elbow or knee, etc., the same applies for the smaller joints such as your fingers and the vertebrae that make up your spine. This lubricating system is near perfect—it is designed *not* to wear out. And yet we see that it actually does! Why would that be?

Historically, arthritis has always been regarded as a very common and slowly progressive disorder, that is most often seen in the elderly, and which affects all the weight-bearing joints such as knees, hips, the spine, etc. It has been thought and generally accepted that it is an integral part of aging; that it is usually something you get when you get older. If we believe this line of thinking, how would we explain a ten-year-old having the beginnings of arthritis?

Essentially, osteoarthritis is an enormous, self-contained *remodeling* process. That is the key to understanding what I am about to explain next. It is, in essence, your own body attempting to repair something that has been damaged or changed, or under undue stress; a joint that is under tremendous stress and is beginning to wear down because of that particular stress. When I am speaking of stress here, I am not referring to psychological stress. I am referring to actual physical stress on a particular joint or vertebrae.

The initiating and common denominator in this process of deterioration, which is what arthritis is, is simply an alteration or change in the, what we call, normal bio-mechanical pattern of movement of some of the vertebrae of the spine. In other words, there is a change in the function of some of the individual vertebrae. This change is not seen as something normal, however. It is what we call a patho-biomechanical change – an alteration in normal movement. This is what causes abnormal stress on a particular joint.

What I am referring to here is an example of a *vertebral subluxation*. This can be seen as either a "misalignment" or a change in normal function. As a result, there is considerable "splintering" of the cartilage and the production of what is referred to as "microfractures" of the cartilage of a joint.

When referring to two vertebrae in the spine, which a disc separates, I must mention that the disc also undergoes a number of changes. It tends to decrease in size and fissures form in its material. This tends to lead to instability and as a result, the normal body's repair phenomena are called into play in an attempt to stabilize an area that is unstable. As a result, we see the formation of calcium deposits, bone spurs, etc. These are seen as buttressing mechanisms in order to aid stability. Arthritis is now no longer seen in terms of an actual disease; it is viewed upon as your own body attempting to repair an area of your spine that is unstable. This process can be likened to a snowball rolling down a hill, and gathering not only speed, but also size and weight. The process of arthritis can be broken down into four very distinct stages or phases that actually tend to blend together into a continuous progressive condition.

Let me illustrate what I mean. I am going to use the neck area or cervical spine as an example only because it is much easier to see on x-ray than any other part of the spine. There are a number of characteristics of a normal neck or cervical spine that one can see on a side-view x-ray (lateral view). There are seven vertebrae all arranged in a beautiful synchronized curvature. If I draw a beautiful line across the front of each vertebra with a normal radius of 17 cm, each vertebra should touch this normal cervical arc. The spaces between the vertebra where the discs are located are even, and the edges of the vertebrae are likewise. The corners of the vertebrae are round and smooth and there are no calcium deposits. The openings between the vertebrae where the nerves exit from the spinal cord are also very smooth, round and regular in shape. This is an example of normal.

PHASE I

Phase one is seen as the earliest evidence of arthritis. It is characterized mainly by instability of some of the vertebrae, which then causes weakness throughout the whole area. There is also evidence that there are obvious vertebral subluxations present. As well, the curvature of the spine in that area is generally either lost or actually in the reversed configuration.

PHASE II

This phase is characterized by evidence on x-ray that the discs between the vertebrae are actually smaller than they should be. In other words, the discs are beginning to deteriorate. The edges of the vertebrae are now roughened and we actually begin to see the beginnings of calcium deposits. As well, there is also evidence that the vertebral subluxations have increased in severity. The openings that allow the nerves to pass through from the spinal cord are beginning to be roughened and smaller than they normally should be. This is a problem.

PHASE III

This phase is much more serious and is characterized by advanced and massive calcium deposits, spur formation, the collapse of most of the discs, the onset of deformity of some of the vertebrae, and the beginnings of fusion – not a good thing!

PHASE IV

This last phase is characterized by total loss of form and function of the spine and the vertebrae in that area. There is evidence of bone deformation and total fusion, as well as calcification of most of the spinal ligaments that hold the vertebrae together in that area. Phase four is the condition, which is irreparable.

For a clearer explanation of the above, please ask your family chiropractor as he/she would be happy to explain this in much more detail. As I have mentioned earlier, there has been a general feeling for years that arthritis and all the phases, which have been discussed, is a part of aging. I would like to state that this type of thinking is absolute nonsense. Arthritis is not caused by aging. It is caused by some of the vertebrae in the spine being subluxated while others are perfectly normal.

Consider a case, for example, which a chiropractor would see quite often. This is an example of an individual who has pain perhaps in the back, perhaps leg pain, weakness, numbness and tingling, cramping in the calf, and possible difficulty with bowel function. In most cases, this person would seek the opinion of the family medic who would perform an examination, followed by x-rays, and would discover that the bottom disc of the spine is severely deteriorated while a disc, two or three above that one, would be perfectly normal. This person would then be told that they have arthritis.

How many of you would feel that the two discs I just described, because they belonged to the same person, are most likely the same age? If you said yes, you are then definitely on the ball. If the deterioration of this person's disc was due to age, then the disc above it would look the same. And, in almost every case I have seen at my Centre, there is usually one, or two, or perhaps three that are deteriorating and the rest are quite normal.

The point I am making is that *arthritis has nothing to do with aging*. I repeat, nothing to do with aging. It has to do with the subluxation of the spine, which has never been corrected. I mentioned subluxations occurring during the process of delivery, and this is the reason I very often find the beginning of arthritis in children who are five, six and even ten years old. It is the beginning of the process. If I then saw this particular child as an adult at the age of twenty-five, I would most likely see that same condition much more advanced.

This next bit of news may just brighten up your day. I am very proud to say that a number of years ago, approximately fifty Ontario chiropractors, of which I was part, were involved in a major research study that involved literally thousands of patients. We discovered that if a vertebral subluxation was corrected, it was then possible to not only arrest and stop the process of arthritis, but we actually found that in many cases it could be reversed. Let me repeat this sentence to make sure you got it. *We found that arthritis could be not only slowed down and stopped, but also reversed.* That's profound!

I sat down and decided to write up this research study[80] and have it published. Since that time, it has been proven by other researchers to be the case. My point being is that it is very important to have children checked to determine whether or not they have subluxations. Not only from the perspective of insuring normal health and function of the nervous system, but also to make certain that there is no error in the function of the vertebrae that would then cause this arthritic process we talked about to start.

---

[80] Ressel, O., "Disc Regeneration; Reversibility is Possible in Spinal Osteoarthritis," *ICA Review*, September, 1989.

In October of 2004, I had a sequel to that original research paper published (I mentioned this earlier) where we found that over 85 percent of children demonstrated the beginnings of osteoarthritis. So ... please have your kids checked. There is compelling evidence that this is a very wise thing to do. To make this real for you, allow me to tell you a story.

Years ago, when I was very green at this healing game, I received a frantic call from a young nineteen-year-old girl. She was in severe pain and I was her last resort. Being in practice only a short while at the time, I had this girl come to the office at once and here is her story. She was employed as a teller in a local bank, and would have to get up at 5:00 a.m., because she needed the time to stand in a hot shower and let the hot water run down her back and legs. This was necessary for her to be limber enough to put on her panty hose. Many times she could not walk but had to crawl on her hands and knees! We are talking about a nineteen-year-old here!

By noon, the bank would be forced to send her home because of severe pain. She had frequent reactions to the amounts of aspirin she was taking for pain – there was no Tylenol in those days. She finally went to the family doctor who subsequently sent her for physiotherapy. She went faithfully, three times per week. The pain increased. She was referred to an orthopedic surgeon who couldn't help. She was finally sent to a Rheumatologist, blood tests were done and it was conclusively confirmed that she had Rheumatoid Arthritis. She was told that by the time she reached her twenty-fourth birthday, she would probably be in a wheelchair! Her parents were not wealthy people, having recently emigrated from England, and they were saving money so that they could build ramps around their house for their daughter. These are the circumstances of how I met this girl.

To make a long story short, as I started to correct her subluxations, the pain began to subside, the laboratory tests for rheumatoid arthritis eventually became negative, and as we worked together, we became very close. And that is the story of my wife.

I want you to know that we have no wheelchair at home, Linda is in no pain, and does not have arthritis.

Phases Of Progressive Lumbar Degeneration

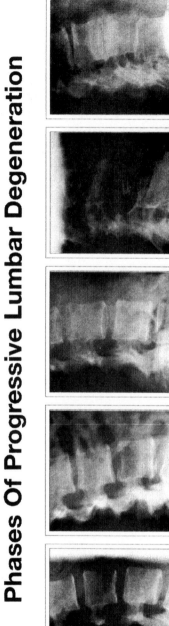
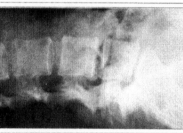

NORMAL SPINE

INCIDENCE:
- diverse

ONSET:
- at birth (also possible after corrective chiropractic care)

HISTOPATHOLOGY AND X-RAY:
- there are no vertebral subluxations
- edges and margins of vertebrae are smooth and regular
- joint surfaces are not roughened and are evenly spaced
- spine exhibits normal lordotic curve
- disc spaces are healthy
- there is no tissue damage

MOST COMMON SYMPTOMS:
- none

CORRECTIVE TIME:
- none required

% OF RECOVERY:
- not applicable

PHASE I

INCIDENCE:
- most often birth - 20 years

ONSET:
- usually a traumatic incident producing vertebral subluxations which remain uncorrected.
- vertebral subluxations produced are an adaptation to a pelvic malfunction.

HISTOPATHOLOGY AND X-RAY:
- vertebral subluxations and disc stress are evident
- nerve pressure resulting in rupture of nerve roots
- liver, pancreas and adsorption into surrounding tissues or loss of subluxation affecting other nerve systems
- normal nerve function is hampered
- can trace loss of normal spine curve
- minimal soft tissue damage at this point

MOST COMMON SYMPTOMS:
- spine stiffness
- occasional "twinges" of pain which seem to "go away"
- low back soreness
- spinal numbness in toes and calves
- leg weakness and fatigue
- cramping in legs thought to be "growing pains"
- occasional gas, bloating, and digestive difficulties
- severe menstrual pains
- abdominal cramps
- fatigue when standing

CORRECTIVE TIME:
- 6 - 18 months

% OF RECOVERY:
- 100%, however dependent on patient compliance

PHASE II

INCIDENCE:
- most often 20 - 40 years

ONSET:
- Phase I, a vertebral subluxation which has not been corrected

HISTOPATHOLOGY AND X-RAY:
- vertebral subluxations increase in severity
- vertebral margins roughen
- joint surfaces become rough and irregular
- abnormal calcium production
- bone spurs are evident at edges of vertebrae
- discs narrow and show signs of degeneration, decay and dehydration
- normal nerve function and transmission not possible
- muscular atrophy and wasting has begun

MOST COMMON SYMPTOMS:
- increasing stiffness, usually in the morning
- numbness and tingling into feet and toes
- low back pain radiating into legs
- groin pains
- abdominal bloating and gas
- constipation (or diarrhea)
- bowel problems
- clumsiness
- reduction of normal reflexes
- "the back that always gives out" syndrome
- tired feeling in the back when standing

CORRECTIVE TIME:
- 18 - 30 months

% OF RECOVERY:
- dependent on severity and patient compliance

PHASE III

INCIDENCE:
- most often 40 - 65 years

ONSET:
- Phase II, a vertebral subluxation which remained uncorrected

HISTOPATHOLOGY AND X-RAY:
- beginnings of bone fusion evident
- abnormal calcium and arthritic formation
- abnormal calcium production
- soft tissue decay very evident
- vertebral deformity started
- disc function in foot and discs are degenerated
- poor nerve function, neurological transmission is seriously impaired
- nerve failure has started
- muscular atrophy and wasting of pelvic and lower limb muscles

MOST COMMON SYMPTOMS:
- constant episodic low back pain (comes and goes)
- greatly reduced movement
- over-all stiffness
- low back pain and fatigue
- increasing back and pelvic problems
- leg and foot pain and/or problems
- numbness in feet and toes
- some inco-ordination when walking
- pain which tends to appear for "no apparent reason"
- urinary difficulties
- digestive difficulties

CORRECTIVE TIME:
- usually 30 - 42 months, however a degree of permanency may remain

% OF RECOVERY:
- dependent on severity and patient compliance

PHASE IV

INCIDENCE:
- most often after 65 years but not always

ONSET:
- Phase III, a vertebral subluxation which were not corrected

HISTOPATHOLOGY AND X-RAY:
- most vertebrae have lost their form and function
- fusion is complete
- spinal form is destroyed
- discs have completely degenerated
- muscular atrophy and utilisation with calcium calcification of most spinal ligaments
- nerve system failure
- nerve transmission is lost
- nerve death and atrophy
- a terminal condition has been created

MOST COMMON SYMPTOMS:
- little movement
- chronic, unremitting pain in most areas
- difficulty in walking
- wasting of most leg muscles
- severe fatigue
- chronic bowel and bladder malfunction
- poor circulation
- numbness
- failure of related organ systems is evident
- untimely death

CORRECTIVE TIME:
- none possible, care at this point for relief and comfort only

% OF RECOVERY:
- none

THE PRACTICE EVOLUTION PROGRAM
PROFESSIONAL DESIGN GROUP
Ottawa, Canada 1-800-363-9082

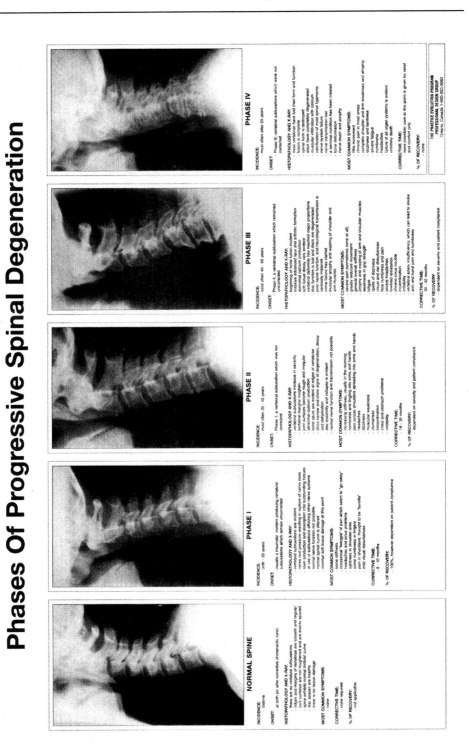

25. Choosing a Chiropractor

Many of you have experienced the excitement of starting chiropractic care, of finally correcting the problems that have caused so many of yours, your family's and children's difficulties, and sharing that experience with your coworkers and family. When sharing your experience with others though, you most likely have come across comments such as; "my chiropractor does not do that" or "my chiropractor only wants to see me when it hurts" or "my chiropractor does not see children." This diversity among the same profession can be very confusing to the average person. But think about this for a moment. Many other professions are also faced with diversity and certain members have special training and expertise. This is quite normal.

There are essentially two distinct types of chiropractors, according to Dr. Patrick Gentempo, a noted lecturer, author, and friend: The *limited scope* chiropractor and the *full spectrum* chiropractor. Let me explain what this means.

The limited scope doctor limits his/her practice to the "treatment" of aches and pains, sports injuries, rehabilitation, motor vehicle injuries and other musculo-skeletal difficulties. This type of practice is essentially "crisis control." Although not wellness-oriented, this type of doctor does, nevertheless, provide a very important function. This type of practice is based on a medical model of health care: a detailed history of symptoms, an orthopaedic examination, (which really does not locate or describe the nature of the subluxation), x-rays (if warranted), and then a diagnosis. This ritual is usually followed by "treatment" of the condition and has little to do with subluxation correction and wellness care. This is the doctor most people think of when they are in pain. So if you have discomfort and only want relief, then this is the type of doctor you should see.

The full spectrum chiropractor, on the other hand, has a different mission – the correction of vertebral subluxations and providing patients

235

with optimal health. Vertebal subluxations interfere with the function of your nervous system and the ability of your body to function normally. If allowed to remain, vertebral subluxations will eventually produce malfunction, which can lead to pathology and disease. Since 85 percent of vertebral subluxation can be the result of Traumatic Birth Syndrome, the full spectrum doctor will suggest that your children and family members be checked for subluxations as soon as possible. This has nothing to do with symptoms or any other health problem your child or member of your family may be experiencing. This type of practice is a wellness practice and involves not only making your body function optimally but also maintaining that level of function. Within these two models, there are chiropractors that have availed themselves of special training, specialty degrees, etc. These can be in fields such as pediatrics, nutrition, research, teaching, athletics, etc.

Let's look at the education of a chiropractor.

There has much confusion among the public regarding chiropractic education. Some heard that it is a three-month course in "cracking" the back. (I know, it sounds horrible to me also.) Others think that it is an apprenticeship, like carpentry. Most people have little idea. Let me set this record straight. A chiropractic student is accepted only after he/she has completed three years of a recognized university program (two years in the United States). This undergraduate work will then entitle an applicant to apply to a chiropractic college, and presently there are twenty-four such colleges around the globe.

In addition to classroom work, there is an intensive two-year internship period where interns look after real patients under the supervision of a licensed clinician. Some may also be involved in an externship program where they may assist field chiropractors in their offices. The majority of schoolwork is done in the classroom and laboratory.

Many people ask how chiropractic education compares to medical education. I'm glad you asked. I'll tell you ... the basic science courses are almost the same – neurology, anatomy, physiology, etc. There are important differences also.

Dr. Tedd Koren, a good friend and author, summarized this comparison in classroom hours on the following table:

Chiropractic		Medicine
540	**Anatomy**	508
240	**Physiology**	326
360	**Chemistry**	401
165	**Pathology**	325
120	**Microbiology**	114
630	**Diagnosis**	324
320	**Neurology**	112
360	**X-Ray**	148
60	**Obstetrics**	148
60	**Psychiatry**	144
210	**Orthopaedics**	156
3,065	**Total Hours**	**2,706**

Other Required Subjects
  Spinal Adjustments   Pharmacology
  Pediatrics   Immunology
  Advanced Radiology   General Surgery

Grand Total Class Hours
  Chiropractic   **4,485**
  Medicine   **4,248**

After completing these requirements, the Intern graduates as a Doctor of Chiropractic and must pass license examinations for Canada and the United States. As well, he must also pass stringent provincial and state examinations before he/she is allowed to practice. There you have it. From my perspective, chiropractic education is tougher than medical school.

In conclusion, there are two types of chiropractors. Which doctor you choose will depend on the type of care you are looking for. Both are here to help you and both are highly trained and educated. So choose wisely.

Epilogue . . . sort of

Well, there you have it.

The pages you have read are but a sprinkle upon a vast ocean of knowledge that is continuously in the process of being updated and refined. It is part of the movement I have mentioned in Chapter 2 – the Paradigm Shift. This shift is unstoppable; those who think that they can stand in its way are suffering from delusions of grandeur. Those who think there is no such force have a serious case of cerebral constipation. They need to be adjusted.

Someone once asked Wayne Gretzky, the Great One, what made him the best. After all, he is not the fastest, not the tallest, not the best looking, why is he then called The Great One? His answer, I'll never forget:

"While everyone is chasing the puck, I am where the puck is going."

Profound!

And so it is with Chiropractic. It is where the health care movement is going. People are beginning to embrace a philosophy of life, a concept of Wellness that the Profession of Chiropractic has been teaching for one-hundred and fifteen years. People like the science, the philosophy, the logic, and the simplicity of the chiropractic approach to health.

It is honest and makes total sense – an unbeatable combination.

I sincerely hope that the words I have put on paper have made you think. I hope they have made you ponder your rationale and approach to the health of your family.

You see, truth is very difficult to put aside. It has that certain quality which touches the very being. It allows you to know innately what you should do. You may choose to resist for a time, but eventually, deep down inside, you will know that it is correct.

Chiropractic - our time has arrived!

Appendix
The Politics of Health

Many people have held the notion (which has been totally supported by organized medicine), that the family physician is of a benevolent nature. He/she will take the best care of you, and maintain the health of your family and your children for the rest of their lives. This seems to be the fable under which many people live out their lives. Unfortunately, as in every other facet of our lives, politics does play an integral part. What a shock!

Did you know, for example, that a number of major studies revealed that breakfast is the most important meal of the day? Just to let you know how prevalent this thinking is, if I suggested that you approach any unsuspecting neighbor and asked them "What is the most important meal of the day?" Their answer would be, "breakfast." You may be wondering "So what, is this important?" Well, maybe it is, and maybe it isn't. It depends on your perspective.

The reason I am stating this question is to simply point out that politics plays a very important role in health. Getting back to our study on breakfast, let me ask you this; have you any idea who this study was funded by? If you guessed that it was the breakfast cereal companies, then you are brilliant! The study was funded and actually conducted by the breakfast cereal makers to promote breakfast cereal. We have been carefully taught to believe that this is absolutely the truth. Now don't get me wrong here, I am not stating that breakfast is not the most important meal of the day. The point I am simply making is that companies who have a financial interest in the results of the study funded the study. This is called "politics" and can be seen in every facet of health care.

Most of you are undoubtedly aware of *The Good Housekeeping Seal of Approval.* It was a label placed on products, and I believe also services, which were recognized and approved of by the American Medical Association in the 1960s, 70s, etc. This seal of approval had very little to do with whether the product or service was beneficial.

Apparently, it was simply, how much money a manufacturer donated to organized medicine to obtain their "blessing." This seal certainly did not provide a consumer with a better product. As I understand, it was simply paid advertising.

Here is another example of "politics at work." On June 30, 2000, my wife and I were driving from Canada to South Carolina for a vacation with our children. At 5:30 A.M., we heard, on a popular Toronto radio station, that the "once-a-day" aspirin habit, (that so many people hold dear to their hearts as a good preventative measure of stroke, heart attack, etc), is actually *not good for you*. As I only caught a portion of the segment, I thought I would listen for later news report to obtain more information. You would be surprised to learn that the broadcast was not repeated. It seems that it was pulled off the air and I can only imagine why.

Let's see ... the manufacturer of aspirin pays out millions of dollars in advertising. Some of that goes to the radio station I just mentioned. I could just imagine the conversation when one of the CEO's of the manufacturing company heard the newscast. Here is the way I think it probably went. "Either you pull this news story or we will pull our ads." Guess who won? Yes, integrity is difficult to find when placed side by side with money. In case you wondered what the story was all about, I thought I would fill you in on the latest talk about aspirin.

The drug companies that make and market aspirin have tried hard to convince the public that, "an aspirin a day, keeps the heart attack away." A recent British study found that it actually does more *harm,* than good. The pharmaceutical industry immediately began a massive press release campaign, which distorted the research study. The press releases gave the impression that daily aspirin was a sure-fire method of preventing heart attacks. Newspapers carried this story and physicians began prescribing aspirin as a preventative measure.

Thanks to this deceptive marketing campaign, North Americans take over 25 million aspirin tablets *everyday,* despite the fact that:

- 1,600 children die each year from allergic reactions to aspirin.
- Patients with blockage of arteries to the brain are three times more likely to have a stroke if they are taking aspirin.
- Indigestion and gastrointestinal hemorrhage occur in 31 percent of those taking 300 mg. of aspirin per day.
- Low doses of aspirin can increase the risk of brain hemorrhage.
- Other side effects include anemia, bleeding ulcers, confusion and dizziness, to name a few.

Can you now guess why this story was not repeated on the air? Let me give you some more examples of the "politics of health" from my own personal experience.

My practice was in Burlington, Ontario, Canada, and, according to my peers, was one of the largest children's and family practices in North America. The College of Chiropractors of Ontario, which is our licensing body and is comparable to a State Board in the United States, and of which I was a Council Member, has a subcommittee called the Chiropractic Review Committee (CRC). Their function is to investigate "unusual" billings to the Provincial Health Plan that pays, in part, for chiropractic care for any resident of Ontario. The Chiropractic Review Committee, acting on orders from The College of Chiropractors of Ontario and the Manager of The Provincial Insurance Plan, decided to investigate my practice a number of years ago.

Apparently, my computer billing profile at the Provincial office showed that I see "too many" children and families; much higher than the "average" Chiropractor, which was considered an "unusual" statistic. Our government keeps profiles of busy and above average doctors and compares these statistics to those who are not so.

Wait...it gets better!

An inspector for the CRC was sent to our Centre and spent several days examining patient records, files, procedures, etc., in other words, every aspect of the daily operation of the Centre. The inspector wrote a glowing report about our practice to the CRC Committee.

Here is where it really gets interesting.

Whoever was in charge probably did not like this type of shining report and so a few weeks later another inspector was sent for a follow-up inspection – a very unusual procedure! As you may have guessed, this new report was totally the opposite: I was seeing too many children, care was not up to standard, the insurance company was billed for too many children, etc. (In retrospect, I now realize that this was an elaborate plan for an economic recovery program and has been enacted with many of the top doctors in the province.)

This latest report made certain that I was called in front of the Review Committee for an "informal interview." The CRC unilaterally decided that I had to repay back to the provincial health care plan the amount of approximately $20,000 for care, which the committee felt was not needed, nor necessary for the children that I cared for. As you can imagine, not only was I shocked and surprised, but I was also very angry. I appealed the Committee's decision to a higher court and after some two years and a four day hearing later, I not only won my appeal in total, but the Court severely admonished the CRC and the College, for what they called a "sloppy presentation."

The reason I have mentioned this particular incident is because the "investigations" of this committee seem nothing more than an economic recovery program by the Province of Ontario to make wrong, high profile practitioners doing honest work – simply not OK!

I won, however, it burned my bridges with the College – imagine that!

Let me share with you another example.

Some 15 years ago or so, approximately 50 chiropractors from the Province of Ontario were involved in a major research study. We found that spinal arthritis, disc degeneration, etc. can actually not only be slowed down and stopped, but that arthritis can actually be reversed in many cases. I must refer you to the initial premise in this book where I mention that the body is a self-healing organism. It is very true that arthritis can be reversed. I wrote our study in a research format, and had the findings peer-reviewed and published in the United States. My own College of Chiropractors of Ontario, the same one mentioned above, decided that it is not possible to cause arthritis to be reversed, and therefore, charged me with misconduct for publishing information which was not true. For those not familiar with this terminology, it is a very serious charge and can cause a health professional to lose his license. A four-year disciplinary hearing followed. Experts were summoned and finally the College admitted defeat. They told me that they were very sorry for pursuing it, no hard feelings and life goes on. There was absolutely no reimbursement for my legal fees, which were sizable, as well as the worry and concern that they caused me, because they felt that they were simply "protecting the public" – their mandate. Nice bunch!

You may find this next bit of information quite eye-opening.

Whenever the College of Chiropractors of Ontario receives a complaint from the public, a complaint about a chiropractor, the College is under mandate to deal with it – even if it is frivolous. (By comparison, the medical licensing body throws out most of the complaints it receives.) The assumption that is generally made is that the person who is complaining is honest, sincere, and the complaint is considered true. Amazing! If that is the case, then the doctor is automatically made to be wrong, no matter what, and must then prove his/her innocence. I know of no court in the land where someone must prove his innocence. On the contrary, people are considered innocent *until* proven guilty. It is the responsibility of the court to prove a person guilty – as it should be. Not our College! It happens the other way.

There's more . . .

Some of the complaints are dismissed and doctors may receive a verbal "caution," which amounts to a reprimand – even if the doctor happens to be right! Other complaints are turned over to a Discipline Committee, which then decides to hold an "informal" conference to see if the complaint warrants a full hearing. Let me place you in the shoes of a doctor called in front of this "informal" pre-trial conference, so you can understand the full meaning behind the scenes.

You, as the doctor, are facing the prosecutor, the representative of the Discipline Committee, the College Registrar, a court reporter and the College's independent attorney and you are trying very hard to understand what they mean by the word "informal." The prosecutor builds his whole case from the complaint and the testimony of "experts" used by the College to destroy the credibility of the doctor and score points. The case is carefully contrived, invented, and manufactured in many cases, to suit their end. The doctor hires a defense attorney, a move that in many cases is hopeless, as the College it seems has already decided what it wants to do and simply steam rolls along. The word justice is given lip service only. Politics and power count.

You, as the Doctor, are then presented with a carefully manu-factured, concocted, and masterminded case against you, which is almost not defensible. The future looks bleak. The College then moves in for the kill. They inform the doctor, who I may add, has not been found guilty of any wrongdoing, and offer to plea-bargain. The doctor is told that the College will accept, as penalty, a suspension of his license to practice, for a specified period of time. In return, they will make the looming trial "go away" saving the doctor tens of thousands, even hundreds of thousands of dollars in legal fees if he pleads *guilty* (even if he is not). Most doctors cannot afford to defend themselves in this manner and against such overwhelming odds and so they capitulate. Right or wrong makes no difference. The College has won and has pleased the government, in that it is doing its job of "protecting the public," and that's what counts. The College can then use this new guilty plea against the doctor in the future. Fair? No. Just? No. Legal? Yes.

Let me share another scenario with you that involves Dr. Joseph Kropf who is a member of the Ontario Medical Association. He has been charged with misconduct for using "treatments" that have not been approved by the Medical Association in Canada; treatments such as herbs, natural health products and so forth. There was a large movement in Canada to collect money across the country to help Dr. Kropf with his battle against the medical licensing body, the College of Physicians and Surgeons of Ontario. He lost.

You may or may not be aware that I wrote for two national magazines and a number of local newspapers, including a pediatric column entitled *Kids First*; this is where the name of the book originated. A few years ago, I started a series of articles in the newspapers dealing with the controversy of vaccination. The local Chief Medical Officer of Health called one such newspaper and had my newspaper columns canceled as being too controversial for the public to read. Yet the information I have presented is well researched, well documented, and true.

The fear of the Chief Medical Officer of Health was that the articles might create free thought in the mind of the public, which could you to believe that perhaps there is more to vaccination than is presented. As a matter of fact, one of my colleagues runs a cable TV show in Brantford, close to Burlington, Ontario where my practice was located. One of his guests was to be Catherine Diodati, Ontario's vaccine researcher, who had just written a number of books on vaccination. The local Chief Medical Officer of Health in his county asked the TV station to cancel the show as being too controversial.

Guess what happened? The show was canceled.

And it goes on ... ad nauseum!

Bibliography

-ADHD Fraud website: http://home.att.net/~fred-alden

-Adkinson, N.F., Jr., Eggleston, P.A., Eney, D., Goldstein, E.P, Schuberth, K.C., Bacon, J.R., Hamilton, R.G., Weiss, M.E., Arshad, H., Meinert, C.L., Tonascia, J., Wheeler, B., A *Controlled trial of immunotherapy for asthma in allergic children,* New Eng. Jnl Med 1997, 336 (5):324-31.

-Alderson, M., *International Mortality Statistics: Facts on File,* (Wash. D.C. 1981), 17-8.

-*Alternative Medicine*, Future Medicine Publishing, Tiburon, CA.

-*America Says No to Ritalin*, Planet Chiropractic, Sept. 15, 2000.

-Andrews, L.B., Stocking, C., Krizek, T., Gottlieb, L., Krizek, C., Vargish, T., Siegler, M., *An alternative strategy for studying adverse events in medical care,* Lancet 1997: 349:309-313.

-Anrig, C., Plaugher G., *Pediatric Chiropractic,* Williams and Wilkins, Baltimore, MD, 1998.

-Anrig-Howe C. *Scientific ramifications for providing prenatal chiropractic care,* The American Chiropractor 1993, May/June 20-3.

-*Autism, is there a vaccine connection?*,Vaccination Risk Awareness Newsletter, March 2000.

-Baguley, D.N.M., Glasgow, G.L., *Subacute sclerosing panencephalitis and the Salk vaccine*, Lancet 1973, 2:763-5.

-Bangle, F., *Idiopathic Scoliosis. Identifiable causes, detection and correction.* Baldwin Brothers, Inc., 2nd edition, 1986.

-Bates, D.W., et al., *The costs of adverse drug events in hospitalizations*, Adverse Drug Events Prevention Study Group, JAMA, 1997; 277(4):307-11.

-Bates, D.W., Spell, N., Cullen, D.J., Burdick, E., Laird, N., Petersen, L.A., Small, S.D., Sweitzer, B.J., Leape, L.L., *The costs of adverse drug events in hospitalized patients,* Adverse Drug Events Prevention Study Group. JAMA 1997, 277(4): 307-11.

-Baughman, F., *Treatment of Attention Deficit Hyperactivity Disorder*, Journal of the American Medical Association, April 28, 1999.

-*Bause, G.S., Niebyl J.R., Sanders R..C., Doppler ultrasound and maternal erythrocyte fragility,* Obstet Gynecol 1983, 62(1):7-10.

-Bell, Rachel, Peiper, H., *The A.D.D. and A.D.H.D. Diet*, Safe Goods, Sheffield, MA, 2006.

-Berman S; *Management of acute otitis media in pediatric practice,* Curr Pediatr 1995, 7(5)513-22.

-Biederman, H., *Kinematic Imbalances Due to Suboccipital Strain in Newborns,* Journal Manual Medicine, 1992; 6:151-156.

-Biederman, H., *Resolution of infantile Erb's palsy utilizing chiropractic treatment,* Jnl Manipulative Physiol Ther 1994, 17(2):129-31.

-Blomerth, P.R., *Functional nocturnal enuresis,* Jnl Manipulative Physiol Ther 1994, 17(4\5)335-8.

-Bloom, A.S., Russell, L.J., Weisskopf, B., Blackerby, J.L., *Methylphenidate-induced delusional disorder in a child with attention deficit disorder with hyperactivity,* Jnl Am Acad Child Adolesc Psychiatry 1988, 27(1):88-89.

-Bourguignon, R., Dangers of Fluoxetine (Prozac), Lancet, January 18, 1997.

-Breggin, P., *Talking Back to Ritalin,* Ingram, 1998.

-Breggin, P., *The War Against Children of Color: Psychiatry Targets Inner-city Youth,* Login Brothers, 1998.

-Brewster, D., *The epidemiology of Haemophilus influenzae invasive disease in Scotland prior to immunisation,* Health Bull (Edinb) 1993, 51:385-93.

-Byers, R.K., *Spinal-cord injuries during birth,* Dev Med Child Neurol 1975, 17(1):103-10.

-Campbell, J.D., Elford, R.W., Brant, R.F., *Case-Control Study of Prenatal Ultrasonography Exposure in Children With Delayed Speech,* Can Med Association Journal, 1993, 149(10):1435-40.

-Cantekin, E.I., McGuire, T.W., Griffith, T.L., *Antimicrobial therapy for otitis media with effusion ('secretory' otitis media),* JAMA 1991, 266(23):3309-17.

-*Certification of poliomyelitis eradication*—The Americas, MMWR 43(39):720-2, 19

-Chaitow, L., *Vaccination and Immunization: Dangers, Delusions, and Alternatives,* C.W. Daniel Co. 1994.

-Chiropractic Awareness Council, Guelph, Ontario.

-Citizens Commission on Human Rights, *Protesters Claim Psychiatry Targets Children for Profit,* May 26, 2000.

-Classen, D., *The public should be told that vaccines may have long term adverse effects,* BMJ, Jan. 16, 1989, 318 (2122):183.

-Classen, D.C., Classe, J.B., *The timing of pediatric immunization and the risk of insulin-dependant diabetes mellitus,* Infections Diseases in Clinical Practice, 1997, 6:449-54.

-Classen, D.C., Pestotnik, S.L., Evans, R.S., Lloyd, J.F., Burke, J.P., Adverse drug events in hospitalized patients. Excess length of stay, extra costs, and attributable mortality. JAMA 1997, 277(4):301-6

-Cohen, R., *The antiobiotic treatment of acute otitis media and sinusitis in children,* Diagn Microbiol Infect Dis. 1997, 27(1-2):35-9.

-Coulter, H., *Vaccination, Social Violence, and Criminality: The Medical Assault on the American Brain,* North Atlantic Books. 190.

-Danbert, R.J., *Scoliosis: biomechanics and raationale for manipulative treatment,* Jnl Manipulative Physiol Ther 1989, 12(1)38-45.

-Diamant, M., et al., *Abuse and timing of use of antibiotics in acute otitis media,* Arch Otolryn, 1974, p/ 226-232.

-Diodati, C., *Immunization: History, Ethics, Law, and Health,* Integral Aspects Inc. 1999.

-*Doctor Visits by Youngsters with ADHD up 90%,* Archives of Pediatric and Adolescent Medicine, 1999, 153:1257-1263.

-*Doctor's strike in Israel may be good for health,* British Medical Journal, June 10, 2000.

-Dokheel, T.M., *An epidemic of childhood diabetes in the United States,* Diabetes Care 1993, 16:1606-11.

-Ehrengut, W., *Neural complications after diphtheria vaccinations and inoculations with diphtheria toxoid-mixed vaccines, Observations on their etiopathogenesis,* Dtsch Med Wochenschr 1986, 111(24):939-42.

-Eisenberg, D., et al, *Unconventional Medicine in the United States. Devalued costs and patterns of use,* New England Journal of Medicine, Jan. 28, 1993, 320 (4) 246-52.

-Ellisman M.H., Palmer D.E., Andre M.P., *Diagnostic levels of ultrasound may disrupt myelination,* Exp Neurol 1987, 98(1):78-92.

-*Environmental tobacco smoke: a hazard to children,* American Academy of Pediatrics Committee on Environmental Health. Pediatrics 1997, 99(4):639-42.

-Ewigman, B.G., Crane, J.P., Frigoleto, F.D., LeFevere M.L., Bain, R.P., McNellis, D., *Effect of prenatal ultrasound screening on perinatal outcome,* New England Journal of Medicine, 1993, 329(12):821-7.

-Fenichel, G.M., *Neurological complications of immunization,* Ann neurol 1982, 12(2):119-28.

-Freed, G.L., Bordley, W.C., Clark, S.J., Konrad, T.R., *Reactions of pediatricians to a new centers for disease control recommendation for universal immunization of infants with hepatitis B vaccine,* Pediatrics 1993, 91(4):699-702.

-Friese, K.H., Kruse, S., Moeller, H., *Acute otitis media in children. Comparison between conventional and homeopathic therapy,* HNO 1996, 44(8):462-6.

-Froehle, R.M., *Ear infection: a retrospective study examining improvement from chiropractic care and analyzing for influencing factors,* Jnl Manipulative Physiol Ther 1996, 19(3):169-77.

-Froom, J., Culpepper, L., Grob, P., Bartelds, A., Bowers, P., Bridges-Webb, C., Grava-Gubins, I., Green, L., Lion, J., Somaini, B., et al, *Diagnosis and antibiotic treatment of acute otitis media: report from International Primary Care Network,* BMJ 1990, 300(6724):582-6.

-Froom, J., Culpepper, L., Jacobs, M., DeMelker, R.A., Green, L.A., van Buchem, L, Grob, P., Heeren, T., *Antimicrobials for acute otitis media? A review from the International Primary Care Network,* BMJ 1997, 315(7100):98-102.

-Fysh, P.N., *Chronic Recurrent otitis media: Case series of five patients with recommendations for case management,* Jnl Clin Chiro Ped 1996, 1(2):6.

-Ganiats, T.G., Bowersox, M.T., Ralph, L.P., *Universal neonatal hepatitis B immunization – are we jumping on the bandwagon too early?* J Fam Pract 1993, 36(2):147-9.

-Gardner, S.G., Bingley, P.J., Sawtell, P.A., Weeks, S., Gale, E.A., *Rising incidence of insulin dependent diabetes in children aged under 5 years in the Oxford region: time trend analysis,* The Bart's-Oxford Study Group, BMJ 1997, 315(7110):713-7.

-Gates, G.A., Wachtendorf, C., Hearne, E.M., Holt, G.R., *Treatment of chronic otitis media with effusion: results of tympanostomy tubes,* Am Jnl Otolaryngol 1985, 6(3):249-53.

-Gemmell, H.A., Jacobson, B.H., *Chiropractic management of enuresis: time-series descriptive design,* Jnl Manipulative Physiol Ther 1989, 12(5):386-9.

-Gentempo, P., Personal communication.

-Glenmulen, J., *The Prozac Backlash*, Simon & Shuster, New York, 2000.

-Gutman, G., *Blocked Atlantal Nerve Syndromes in Babies and Infants,* Manuelle Medizin, 1987, 25, pp. 5-10.

-Hahn, C., Mentis, G., *Profitable Diagnosis: The Psychiatric Labelling and Drugging of Children,* Freedom Magazine.

-Harris, S.L., Wood, K.W., *Resolution of infantile Erb's palsy utilizing chiropractic treatment*, Jnl Manipulative Physiol Ther 1993, 16(6), 415-8.

-Harvard Medical School, *Media coverage of new drugs is often misleading*, New England Journal of Medicine, June 1, 2000.

-Horowitz, L. *Emerging Viruses: Aids and Ebola - Nature, Accident or Intentional?* Tetrahedron Publishing, 1996.

-Hviid, C., *A comparison of the effect of chiropractic treatment on respiratory function in patients with respiratory distress symptoms and patients without*, Bull Eur Chiro Union 1978, 26:17-34.

-ICA News Brief, Sept/Oct. 1989, Associated Press wire service.

-International Chiropractic Pediatric Association Newsletters.

-*Is Ritalin Ruling the classroom?*, ABC News commentary, Sept. 20, 2000.

-Jacobson, V., Nielsen, C., Buch, D., Shields, W.D., Christenson, P., Zachau-Christiansen, B., Cherry, J.D., *Relationship of pertussis immunization to the onset of epilepsy, febrile convulsions and central nervous system infections: a retrospective epidemiologic study,* Tokai Jnl Exp Clin Med 1988, 13:137-42.

-Johnson, et al, JAMA, 1997.

-Johnson, J., et al., *Drug related morbidity and mortality – a cost-of-illness model*, Arch Internal Medicine, 1995, 155(18) 1949-56.

-Joncas, J.H., *Preventing the congenital rubella syndrome by vaccinating women at risk*, Can Med. Assoc. Jnl 1983, 129(2):100-2.

Kemp, T., Pearce, N., Fitzharris, P., Crane, J., Fergusson, D., St. George, I, Wickens, K., Beasley, R., *Is infant immunization a risk factor for childhood asthma or allergy?* Epidemiology 1997, 8(6): 678-80.

Kent, Christopher, The Chiropractic Journal, October, 1999.

Klougart, N., Nilsson, N., Jacobsen, J., *Infantile colic treated by chiropractors: a prospective study of 316 cases,* Jnl Manipulative Physiol Ther 1989, 12(4): 281-8.

Koren, T., *Chiropractic; Bringing out the Best in You.*, Koren Publications, Philadelphia, PA, 1997.

Kyle, W.S., *Simian retroviruses, polio vaccine, and origin of AIDS,* Lancet 1992, 339(8739):600-1.

Landrigan, P.J., Witte, J.J., *Neurologic disorders following live measles-virus vaccination*, JAMA 1973, 223(13):1459-62.

Lazarou, J., Pomeranz, B.H., Corey, P.N., *Incidence of adverse drug reactions in hospitalized patients: A meta-analysis of prospective studies,* JAMA 1998, 279(15):1200-1205.

Leads, L., *Error in Medicine,* Journal of the American Medical Association, 1994, 272 (23) p. 1851-7.

Lebour, C., Brown, P., Herman, A., Leembruggen, K., Walton, D., Crisp, T.C., *Chiropractic care of children with nocturnal enuresis: a prospective outcome study,* Jnl Manipulative Physiol Ther 1991, 14(2):110-5.

LeFever, Gretchen, et al., *The Extent of Drug Therapy for Attention Deficit Hyperactivity Disorder among Children in Public Schools,* American Journal of Public Health, 1999, Vol 89, No. 9.

Lesar, T.S., Briceland, L., Stein, D.S., *Factors related to errors in medication prescribing,* JAMA 1997, 277(4):312-7.

Liebeskind D., Bases R., Mendez F., Elequin F., Koenigsberg M., *Sister chromatid exchanges in human lymphocytes after exposure to diagnostic ultrasound,* Science 1979, 205(4412):1273-5.

Liebeskind, D., Bases, R., Elequin, F., Neubort, S., Leifer, R., Goldberg, R., Koenigsberg, M., *Diagostic ultrasound: effects on the DNA and growth patterns of animal cells,* Radiology 1979, 131(1):177-84.

Loe-Fisher, B., *A Shot in the Dark,* National Vaccine Information Centre, Vienna, Virginia.

Loe-Fisher, B., *The Consumers Guide To Childhood Vaccines,* NVIC, Virginia.

-Markowitz, L.E., Preblud, S.R., Orenstein, W.A., Rovira, E.Z., Adams N.C., Hawkins, C.E., Hinman, A.R., *Patterns of transmission in measles outbreaks in the United States 1985-86,* New Eng Jnl Med 1989, 329(2):75-81.

-Mendelsohn, R., *How to raise a Healthy Child In Spite of Your Doctor,* Contemporary Books, 1984.

-Mendelsohn, R., *The Medical Heretic,* Contemporary Books, 1979.

-Michigan Chiropractic Association.

-Miller, N., *Immunizations: The People Speak Out,* New Atlantean Press 1996.

-Miller, N., *Vaccines: Are They Really Safe and Effective?* New Atlantean Press, 1994.

-Naeye, R.L, *Brain-stem and adrenal abnormalities in the sudden-infant death syndrome,* Am J Clin Pathol 1976, 666(3):526-30.

-Naeye, R.L., Ladis, B., Drage, J.S., *Sudden infant death syndrome. A prospective study,* Am J Dis Child, 1976, 130(11):1207-10.

-National Health Promotion and Disease Prevention Objective, *Conference Criticism: Summary US Dept. of Health and Human Services,* Healthy People 2000, Public Health Services.

-Neustaedter, R., *The Vaccine Guide: Making an Informed Choice,* North Atlantic Books 1997.
-Nilsson, N., Christianson, B., *Prognostic factors in bronchial asthma in chiropractic practice,* J Aust Chiropr Assoc 1988, 18(3):85-7.
-Nilsson, N., *Infant colic and chiropractic,* Eur Jnl Chiropr 1985, 33(4): 264-65.
-Nkowane, B.M., Bart, S.W., Orenstein, W.a., Baltier, M., *Measles outbreak in a vaccinted school population: Epidemiology, chains of transmission and the role of vaccine failures,* Am Jnl Public Health 1987, 77(4): 434-8.
-O'Meara, K., *Doping Kids,* www.insightmag.com/archive.investiga/ aspec11.html.
-Odent, M.R., Culpin, E.E., Kimmel, T., *Pertussis vaccination and asthma: is there a link?* JAMA 1994, 272(8):592-3.
-Olson, A.L., Klein, S.W., Charney, E., MacWhinney, J.B. Jr., McInerny, T.K., Miller, R.L., Nazarian, L.F., Cunningham, D., *Prevention and therapy of serious otitis media by oral decongestant, a double-blind study in pediatric practice,* Pediatrics 1978, 61:679-84.
-Osterholm, M.T., Rambeck, J.H., White, K.E., Jacobs, J.L, Pierson, L.M., Neaton, J.D., Hedberg, C.W., MacDonald, K.L., Granoff, D.M., *Lack of efficacy of haemophilus B polysaccharide vaccine in Minnesota*, JAMA 1988, 260(10):1423-8.
-Pediatrics Academic Societies Annual Conference, JAMA, May 1999, Vol. 281, No. 20.
-PEW Environmental Health Commission, John Hopkins School of Public Health, Reuters Health, May 17, 2000.
-Phillips, D.P., et al, *Increases in US Medication – Error Deaths between 1981 and 1993*, Lancet Letter, 1999, 351 (9103): 643.
-Poliomyelitis – United States, Centers for Disease Control, MMWR 1986, 35:180-2.
-Pulhar, G.R., Schobert, P.D., *Vertebral subluxation and colic: A case study,* Jnl Chiro Research and Clin Invest 1991, 7(3): 75-6.
-Ramazanov, Z., Del Mar Bernal Suarez, M., *Effective natural Stress and Weight Management*, ATN/Safe Goods, E. Canaan CT, 1999.
-Recommended Childhood Immunization Schedule – United States, MMWR 1997, 46(2): 35-40.
-Reed, W.R., Beavers, S., Reddy, S.K., Kern, G., *Chiropractic management of primary nocturnal enuresis,* Jnl Manipulative Physiol Ther 1994, 17(9): 596-600.

-Ressel, O., *Chiropractic and Children; A Rationale for Care*, ICA Review, 1986.

-Ressel, O., *Disc Regeneration – Reversibility is possible in Spinal Osteoarthritis*, ICA Review, 1989.

-Roark R; Berman S., *Continuous twice daily or one daily amoxicillin prophylaxis compared with placebo for children with recurrent acute otitis media,* Pediatr Infect Dis J 1997, 16(4):376-81.

-Rondberg, T., "Ritalin," *Overprescribed and Dangerous*, Health Watch, Chandler, AZ.Vol 4, No. 8.

-Rorrester J., *Chiropractic management of third trimester in-utero constraint,* Can Chiropr 1997, 2(3):8-13.

-Ruck, A., *The lethal dangers of the billion dollar vaccine business*, Money Magazine, Dec., 1996.

-Rushton, J., *SSRI use common in children*, JAMA, May 28, 1999, Vol 281 No. 20.

-Sachis P.N., Armstrong D.L., Becker L.E., Bryan A.C., *The vague nerve and sudden infant death syndrome: a morphometric study,* J Pediatr 1981, 98(2):278-80.

-Satterfield, J.H., Satterfield, B.T., Schell, A.M., *Therapeutic interventions to prevent delinquency in hyperactive boys*, Jnl Am Acad Child Adolesc Psychiatry 1987, 26(1):56-64.

-Scheibner, V., Ph.D., *Immunizations: 100 Years of Orthodox Research Shows that Vaccines Represent a Medical Assault on the Immune System,* New Atlantean Pr. December 1993.

-Schlafly, Roger, Ph.D., *Official Vaccine Policy Flawed*, Medical Sentinel.

-Schneier M; Burns, R.E., *Atlanto-occipital hypermobility in sudden infant death syndrome.* J Chiropractic Research Clin Invest 1991, 7(2):33.

-Sears, M.R., Taylor, D.R., Print, C.G., Lake, D.C., Li, Q.Q., Flannery, E.M., Yates, D.M., Lucas, M.K., Herbison, G.P., *Regular inha\ed beta-agonist treatment in bronchial asthma,* Lancet 1990, 336:1391-6.

-Shaw, F.E., Jr., Graham, D.J., Guess, H.A., Milstein, J.B., Johnson, J.M., Schatz, G.C., Hadler, S.C., Kuritsky, J.N., Hiner, E.E., Bregman, D.J., et al; *Postmarking surveillance for neurologic adverse events reported after hepatitis B vaccination. Experience of the first three years,* Am Jnl Epidemiol 1988, 127(2), 337-52.

-Smith, R., *Where is The Wisdom–the Poverty of Medical Evidence*, British Medical Journal, Oct. 5, 1991, 303(6806): 798-99.

-Stark, C.R., Orleans, M., Haverkamp, A.D., Murphy, J., *Short and long-term risks after exposure to diagnostic ultrasound in utero,* Obstet Gynecol 1984, 63(2):194-200.

-Statement of the Association of American Physicians And Surgeons to US House of Representatives, Title Subcommittee on Criminal Justice Drug Policy and Human Resources of the Committee on Government Reform.

-Steinschneider, A., *Sudden infant death syndrome and prolongation of the QT interval,* Am Jnl Dis Child 1978, 132(7):688-91.

-Strebel, P.M., Sutter, R.W., Cochi, S.L, Biellik, R.J., Brink, E.W., Kew, O.M., Pallansch, M.A., Orenstein, W.A., Hinman, A.R., *Epidemiology of poliomyelitis in the United States one decade after the last reported case of indigenous wild virus-associated disease,* Clin Infect Dis 1992 , 143(2):568-79.

-Tanchsu P.I., et al., *Scoliosis in Rhythmic Gymnasts,* Spine Journal, 2000, 25 (11): 1367.

-Terracciano, G., Chen, R., Lloyd, J., *Surveillance for Adverse Events Following Vaccination,* CDC Publications 1994.

-Tilyar, M.W., Dovey, S.M., Walker, S.A., *Otitis media treatment in New Zealand general practice,* N Z Med J 1997, 110(1042):143-5.

-Towbin, A., *Latent Spinal Cord and Brain Stem Injury in Newborn Infants,* Medical Child Neurology, 1969, 11, pp. 54-68.

-Tuomilehto, J., Virtala, E., Karvonen, M., Lounamaa, R., Pitkaniemi, J., Reunanen, A., Tuomilehto-Wolf, E., Toivanen, L., *Increase in incidence of insulin-dependent diabetes mellitus among children in Finland,* Int Jnl Epidemiol 1995, 24(5):984-92.

-Van Buchem, F.L., et. al., *Therapy of Acute Otitis Media: Myringotomy Antibiotics, or neither,* Lancet, Oct. 24, 1981, P. 883-887.

-Van Schayck, C.P., Dompeling, E., Van Herwaarden, C.L., Folgering, H., Verbeek, A.L., Van der Hoogen, H.J, Van Weel, C., *Bronchodilator treatment in moderate asthma or chronic bronchitis: continuous or on demand? A randomised controlled study,* BMJ 1991,
303:1426-31.

-Veldhuizem, A.G., et al., *The Autiology of Idiopathic Biomechanical and Neuromuscular Factors,* European Spine Journal, 2000, 9:178.

-Virtanen, H., *Eustachian tube function in children with secretory otitis media,* Int Jnl Pediatr Otorhinolaryngol 1983, 5(1):11-7.

-Walene, J., *Mass Immunization: The Reality behind the Myth,* Bergin & Harvey 1988.
-Ward, J., Brenneman, G., Letson, G.W., Heyward, W.L., *Limited efficacy of a haemophilus influenzae type B conjugate vaccine in Alaska native infants,* The Alaskaa H. Influenzae Vaccine Study group. New England Jnl Med 1990, 323(20):1393-1401.
-Ward, J.I., Broome, C.V., Harrison, L.H., Shinefield, H., Black, S., *Haemophilus influenzae type B vaccines: lessons for the future,* Pediatrics 1988, 81(6):886-93.
-Weiner, H., *The Dark side of Immunizations*, Science News, 1997.
-Weiner, L.P., Herndon, R.M., Narayan, O., Johnson, R.T., *Further studies of a simian virus 40-like virus isolated from human brain* J Virol 1972, 10(1): 147-9.
-White, F., *Measles vaccine associated encephalitis in Canada,* Lancet 1983, 2(8351)683.
-Wiseman, B., *Protesters Claim Psychiatry Targets Children for Profit, Citizens Commission on Human Rights*, May 26, 2000.
-Wiseman, B., *Psychiatry. The Ultimate Betrayal*, The Citizens Commission on Human Rights. Los Angeles, CA.
-Yekutiel M, Robin ,G.C., Yarom, R., *Proprioceptive function in children with adolescent idiopathic scoliosis,* Spine 1981, 6(6):560-6.
Studdert David, Mello Michelle, Financial Conflicts of Interest in Physicians' Relationships with the Pharmaceutical Industry – Self-Regulation in the Shadow of Federal Prosecution, N Eng J Med Oct 28, 2004

About the Author

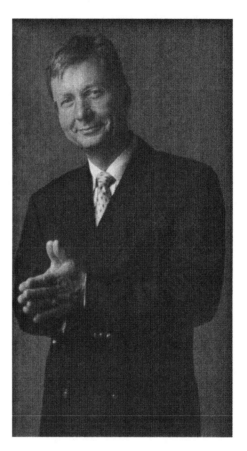

Dr. Ogi Ressel

Dr. Ogi Ressel was a staff writer for *Alive* and *Canada's Healthy Living Guide* magazines, and writes a pediatric column in a number of newspapers in Canada and the US. His writing style is very provocative yet entertaining at the same time. He is also a researcher, lecturer, as well as a pediatric and an x-ray expert. He owned one of the largest children's and family centers in North America. As well, he is a husband, and father of three wonderful, unsubluxated, unvaccinated, healthy children, and resides in Niagara-on-the-Lake, Ontario, Canada.

Index

M

Marketing, 120
Measles, 197, 198, 255, 258
Medical malpractice, 18
Mortality, 249

N

Nature, 57, 63, 253
Nocturnal Enuresis, 119

O

Oppositional Defiant Disorder, 182
Osteoarthritis, 226, 230, 256
Otitis Media, 113, 257

P

Pathology, 237
PM, 67
Polio, 131
Politics, 246
Prozac, 31, 171, 179, 181, 182, 250, 252

R

Registrar, 246
Ritalin, 64, 95, 171, 172, 174, 175, 176, 177, 178, 179, 180, 181, 186, 249, 250, 253, 256

S

Scoliosis, 139, 141, 249, 251, 257

Severe Emotional Disability, 182
Sick, 122
SIDS, 85
SSRI, 181, 256
SV40, 199
Synaptic transmission, 42

T

Traumatic Birth Syndrome, 83, 84, 85, 86, 236

U

Ulcerative Colitis, 147, 148, 149

V

Vaccination, 132, 193, 195, 196, 197, 198, 202, 220, 223, 249, 250, 251, 257
Vacuum extraction, 88
VAERS, 196
Valium, 175
Vertebral Subluxation, 42, 83, 84, 91, 138
Vitamin, 63
VRAN, 202

W

Wellness, 8, 10, 37, 66, 71, 117, 134, 135, 151, 239